Pocket Guide to Kidney Stone Prevention

Manoj Monga
Kristina L. Penniston
David S. Goldfarb
Editors

Pocket Guide to Kidney Stone Prevention

Dietary and Medical Therapy

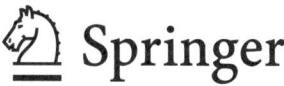

Editors
Manoj Monga, MD, FACS
Stevan Streem Center for
  Endourology & Stone Disease
The Cleveland Clinic
Cleveland, OH, USA

David S. Goldfarb, MD, FACP, FASN
Nephrology Division
NYU Langone Medical Center
New York, NY, USA

Kristina L. Penniston, PhD, RD
Department of Urology
University of Wisconsin School
  of Medicine and Public
  Health
Madison, WI, USA

ISBN 978-3-319-11097-4   ISBN 978-3-319-11098-1 (eBook)
DOI 10.1007/978-3-319-11098-1
Springer Cham Heidelberg New York Dordrecht London

Library of Congress Control Number: 2014952903

© Springer International Publishing Switzerland 2015
This work is subject to copyright. All rights are reserved by the Publisher, whether the whole or part of the material is concerned, specifically the rights of translation, reprinting, reuse of illustrations, recitation, broadcasting, reproduction on microfilms or in any other physical way, and transmission or information storage and retrieval, electronic adaptation, computer software, or by similar or dissimilar methodology now known or hereafter developed. Exempted from this legal reservation are brief excerpts in connection with reviews or scholarly analysis or material supplied specifically for the purpose of being entered and executed on a computer system, for exclusive use by the purchaser of the work. Duplication of this publication or parts thereof is permitted only under the provisions of the Copyright Law of the Publisher's location, in its current version, and permission for use must always be obtained from Springer. Permissions for use may be obtained through RightsLink at the Copyright Clearance Center. Violations are liable to prosecution under the respective Copyright Law.
The use of general descriptive names, registered names, trademarks, service marks, etc. in this publication does not imply, even in the absence of a specific statement, that such names are exempt from the relevant protective laws and regulations and therefore free for general use.
While the advice and information in this book are believed to be true and accurate at the date of publication, neither the authors nor the editors nor the publisher can accept any legal responsibility for any errors or omissions that may be made. The publisher makes no warranty, express or implied, with respect to the material contained herein.

Printed on acid-free paper

Springer is part of Springer Science+Business Media (www.springer.com)

To our patients

Preface

Kidney stones place a heavy burden on physicians and society but most importantly they significantly impact our patients' quality of life. Those who have a first stone attack are highly motivated to make changes to try to avoid recurrence, yet unfortunately only the minority receive appropriate evaluation and counseling.

This handbook was designed to provide the evidence-based tools to make patient-centered recommendations that can decrease the risk of stone recurrence and improve quality of life. We hope you and your patients find it helpful.

Cleveland, OH, USA　　　　　　　　　　　　　　Manoj Monga
Madison, WI, USA　　　　　　　　　　　Kristina L. Penniston
New York, NY, USA　　　　　　　　　　　　David S. Goldfarb

Contents

Part I Counseling the First Time Stone Former

1 What Is the Risk of Stone Recurrence? 3
   Juan C. Calle

2 General Nutrition Guidelines
   for All Stone Formers 9
   Margaret Wertheim

3 24-Hour Urine and Serum Tests:
   When and What? 19
   R. Allan Jhagroo

Part II Calcium Stones
Section 1 *Hypercalciuria*

4 Nutrition Management of Hypercalciuria 29
   E. Susannah Southern

5 Medical Management of Hypercalciuria 37
   Sushant R. Taksande and Anna L. Zisman

Section 2 *Hypocitraturia*

6 Nutrition Management of Hypocitraturia 49
   Liz Weinandy

7 Medical Management of Hypocitraturia 55
   Cynthia Denu-Ciocca

Section 3 *Hyperoxaluria*

8 Nutritional Management of Hyperoxaluria............... 63
Kristina L. Penniston

Part III Uric Acid Stones

9 Nutrition Management of Uric Acid Stones............. 75
Lisa A. Davis

10 Medical Management of Uric Acid Stones................ 81
John S. Rodman

Part IV Cystine Stones

11 Cystinuria... 91
Michelle A. Baum

Part V Struvite Stones

12 Struvite Stones, Diet and Medications 101
Ben H. Chew, Ryan Flannigan, and Dirk Lange

Part VI Follow-Up of the Recurrent Stone Former

13 Laboratory Follow-Up of the Recurrent Stone Former.. 113
Sutchin R. Patel

14 Imaging (Cost, Radiation).. 123
Michael E. Lipkin

15 What to Do About Asymptomatic Calculi................. 131
Shubha De and Sri Sivalingam

Part VII Managing Recurrence

**16 Acute Renal Colic and Medical
 Expulsive Therapy**.. 139
Charles D. Scales Jr. and Eugene G. Cone

17 Stratifying Surgical Therapy... 149
Vincent G. Bird, Benjamin K. Canales,
and John M. Shields

Index... 161

Contributors

Michelle A. Baum, MD Division of Nephrology, Boston Children's Hospital/Harvard Medical School, Boston, MA, USA

Vincent G. Bird, MD Department of Urology, University of Florida College of Medicine, Gainesville, FL, USA

Juan C. Calle, MD Department of Nephrology and Hypertension, Cleveland Clinic, Cleveland, OH, USA

Benjamin K. Canales, MD Department of Urology, University of Florida College of Medicine, Gainesville, FL, USA

Ben H. Chew, MD, MSc, FRCSC Department of Urological Sciences, University of British Columbia, Vancouver, BC, Canada

Eugene G. Cone, MD Division of Urologic Surgery, Duke University Medical Center, Durham, NC, USA

Lisa A. Davis, MS, RD Clinical Research Unit, University of Wisconsin Institute for Clinical and Translational Research, Clinical Science Center, Madison, WI, USA

Shubha De, MD, FRCPC Cleveland Clinic, Glickman Urological and Kidney Institute, Cleveland, OH, USA

Cynthia Denu-Ciocca, MD Kidney Center, University of North Carolina at Chapel Hill, Chapel Hill, NC, USA

Ryan Flannigan, MD Department of Urologic Sciences, University of British Columbia, Vancouver, BC, Canada

R. Allan Jhagroo, MD Department of Medicine and Urology, University of Wisconsin Madison, Madison, WI, USA

Dirk Lange, MD Department of Urologic Sciences, University of British Columbia, Vancouver, BC, Canada

Michael E. Lipkin, MD Division of Urology, Surgery, Duke University Medical Center, Durham, NC, USA

Sutchin R. Patel, MD Department of Urology, University of Wisconsin, School of Medicine and Public Health, Gurnee, IL, USA

Kristina L. Penniston, PhD, RD Department of Urology, University of Wisconsin, School of Medicine and Public Health, Madison, WI, USA

John S. Rodman, MD Department of Medicine/Nephrology, Weill Cornell School of Medicines, New York, NY, USA

Charles D. Scales Jr., MD, MSHS Division of Urologic Surgery, Duke University Medical Center, Durham, NC, USA

John M. Shields, MD Department of Urology, University of Florida College of Medicine, Gainesville, FL, USA

Sri Sivalingam, MD, MSC, FRCSC Cleveland Clinic, Glickman Urological and Kidney Institute, Cleveland, OH, USA

E. Susannah Southern, RDN, LDN Department of Nutrition & Food Services, UNC Health Care, UNC Outpatient Nutrition Clinic, Aycock Family Medicine, Chapel Hill, NC, USA

Sushant R. Taksande, MD Department of Medicine/Section of Nephrology, Pritzker School of Medicine, University of Chicago, Chicago, IL, USA

Liz Weinandy, MPH, RD, LD Nutrition Services, Ohio State University Wexner Medical Center, Dublin, OH, USA

Margaret Wertheim, MS, RD Department of Urology, University of Wisconsin Madison, Madison, WI, USA

Anna L. Zisman, MD Department of Medicine/Section of Nephrology, Pritzker School of Medicine, University of Chicago, Chicago, IL, USA

Part I
Counseling the First Time Stone Former

Chapter 1
What Is the Risk of Stone Recurrence?

Juan C. Calle

On average, it is estimated that 1 in 11 Americans will suffer at least one episode of nephrolithiasis in their life time according to the most recent report from a cross-sectional analysis of large epidemiologic data from the National Health and Nutrition Examination Survey (NHANES) 2007–2010. These data clearly show an increase in the incidence and prevalence of the disease when compared to previous reports from the same database from the period between 1976 and 1980. Multiple factors including changes in diet and lifestyle, increasing epidemics of obesity and diabetes, migration from rural cooler settings to warmer urban areas, and even possibly changes in the global environment with warmer temperatures may all be contributing to this increase in kidney stones [1].

The risk of recurrence after a first kidney stone remains controversial. As early as 1919, Dr. Lamson in a speech before the Association of Residents and Ex-Residents of the Mayo Clinic mentioned a very wide rate of recurrence ranging from 10 to 48 % [2]. Nowadays, reported frequencies of kidney stone recurrence after a first episode range from 30 to 50 % at 5 years in uncontrolled studies and as much as 100 %

J.C. Calle, MD (✉)
Department of Nephrology and Hypertension, Cleveland Clinic, 9500 Euclid Avenue, Cleveland, OH 44195, USA
e-mail: callej@ccf.org

recurrence in patients who form single stones if they were followed for longer than 25 years [3]. These data indicate the complex and heterogeneous natural history of nephrolithiasis. However, recent data from control groups in randomized, controlled trials suggest much lower rates, ranging from 2 to 5 % per year. The risk of recurrence increases with each new stone formed [4]. Therefore, the importance of prevention and assessment of the risk of stone recurrence is highly relevant to any patient and health care provider involved in their care, in particular for those patients with more complex and severe disease.

Some risk factors for stone recurrence cannot be modified; examples include gender, age, family history, gastrointestinal diseases that impact fluid balance and electrolytes, genetic conditions or urologic issues such as medullary sponge kidney or horseshoe kidneys. Other endocrine diseases, mainly related to management of calcium and phosphorus, such as primary hyperparathyroidism, may be modified and treatable [5].

Other independent factors that may increase the chances of recurrence as high as 10 % per year include a history of multiple relapses, increased levels of alkaline phosphatase, stones located in lower calyces as compared to the renal pelvis, multiple stones, stone size larger than 20 mm and younger age. The type of surgical treatment for the first stone event may also influence the recurrence rate and is an active field for research, although many confounding variables make retrospective observations inconclusive [6].

Although metabolic work-up and its possible effect to lower the risk of stone recurrence has not been thoroughly demonstrated, some individuals may benefit from counseling and management based on these results. Metabolic evaluation should then be offered specifically to patients with multiple stones or first stones among complicated cases, in single kidneys, transplant recipients, patients with known severe associated co-morbid conditions, and interested first-time formers [7].

Perhaps the most important aspect of the metabolic work-up is the volume collected during the 24 h collection. Lower urinary volumes have been recognized as a prominent risk factor for recurrence of kidney stones as demonstrated by a well-conducted study by Borghi et al. [8]. Hypercalciuria is the most common abnormality found in patients with kidney stones and urine metabolic work-up other than low fluid intake and low urinary output [9].

Calcium oxalate stones remain as the most common type of kidney stone. Though 24-h urine collections are often used to direct preventive strategies, the values of individual variables at which the risk of recurrence increases are poorly defined. For hyperoxaluria, even small increased levels, generally considered normal (e.g., 25 mg/day) have been shown to put patients at higher risk for formation of stones [10]. Similarly, though hyperuricosuria promotes calcium oxalate stone formation, and medical therapy directed at decreasing urinary uric acid decrease stone recurrence [11], the actual amount of urinary uric acid that increases risk and the role of uric acid in the formation of calcium oxalate stones remains to be elucidated [10].

Urinary citrate plays a role as an endogenous inhibitor of kidney stones by formation of a nondissociable but soluble complex with calcium, hence, decreasing the availability of the calcium to bind with oxalate or phosphate and form crystals. Hypocitraturia, which may happen as an isolated event or in association with other abnormalities also plays an important role as a risk factor for recurrence of kidney stones [12].

As mentioned previously in this chapter, each of these risk factors or components may individually increase the risk of stone recurrence; however, it seems they may all be interconnected, reflected by calculations of supersaturation that have been shown to directly correlate with the formation of kidney stones and subsequent recurrence of the disease. This predictive ability was shown in a large retrospective study by Parks et al. in which patients followed for up to two decades in a specialized kidney stone clinic had less recurrence of stones. This result seemed to be directly correlated with lower levels of supersaturation, at least for those forming calcium oxalate stones [13]. Even though this result has not been confirmed yet in large, randomized control studies, the goal of treatment and management of stone prevention should be targeted towards normalization or improvement of supersaturation as it is recommended in the most recent American Urological Association Guidelines for the medical management of kidney stones [14].

Due to the high recurrence of the disease, multiple co-morbid associations, its impact on quality of life, and the costs directly and indirectly associated with it, kidney stones should be considered a chronic illness that requires long-term advice and management by qualified health care providers with expertise and experience in the subject. Research regarding prevention to decrease the number of relapses is largely and desperately needed.

References

1. Scales Jr CD, Smith AC, Hanley JM, Saigal CS. Urologic diseases in America project. Prevalence of kidney stones in the United States. Eur Urol. 2012;62(1):160–5.
2. Lamson OF. Recurrent nephrolithiasis. Ann Surg. 1920;71(1):16–21.
3. Coe FL, Keck J, Norton ER. The natural history of calcium urolithiasis. JAMA. 1977;238(14):1519–23.
4. Borghi L, Schianchi T, Meschi T, Guerra A, Allegri F, Maggiore U, et al. Comparison of two diets for the prevention of recurrent stones in idiopathic hypercalciuria. N Engl J Med. 2002;346:77–84.
5. Worcester EM, Coe FL. Clinical practice. Calcium kidney stones. N Engl J Med. 2010;363(10):954–63.
6. Chongruksut W, Lojanapiwat B, Tawichasri C, Paichitvichean S, Euathrongchit J, Ayudhya VC, et al. Predictors for kidney stones recurrence following extracorporeal shock wave lithotripsy (ESWL) or percutaneous nephrolithotomy (PCNL). J Med Assoc Thai. 2012;95(3):342–8.
7. Calle JC, Monga M. Metabolic evaluation: underuse or overdone? In: Practical controversies in medical management of stone disease. New York: Springer Science+Business Media; 2014. p. 1–6.
8. Borghi L, Meschi T, Amato F, Briganti A, Novarini A, Giannini A. Urinary volume, water and recurrences in idiopathic calcium nephrolithiasis: a 5-year randomized prospective study. J Urol. 1996;155(3):839–43.

9. Curhan GC, Willett WC, Speizer FE, Stampfer MJ. Twenty-four-hour urine chemistries and the risk of kidney stones among women and men. Kidney Int. 2001;59(6):2290–8.
10. Curhan GC, Taylor EN. 24-h uric acid excretion and the risk of kidney stones. Kidney Int. 2008;73(4):489.
11. Ettinger B, Tang A, Citron JT, Livermore B, Williams T. Randomized trial of allopurinol in the prevention of calcium oxalate calculi. N Engl J Med. 1986;315(22):1386.
12. Parks JH, Coe FL. A urinary calcium-citrate index for the evaluation of nephrolithiasis. Kidney Int. 1986;30(1):85.
13. Parks JH, Coe FL. Evidence for durable kidney stone prevention over several decades. BJU Int. 2009;103(9):1238–46.
14. Pearle MS, Goldfarb DS, Assimos DG, Curhan G, Denu-Ciocca CJ, Matlaga BR, et al. Medical management of kidney stones: AUA guideline. J Urol. 2014;192(2):316–24.

Chapter 2
General Nutrition Guidelines for All Stone Formers

Margaret Wertheim

There are multiple nutritional influences on kidney stone risk, regardless of stone type. These factors include energy balance as it relates to body composition, fluid intake, sodium intake, purine intake from animal flesh, and the acid load of the diet. A 24-h urine collection is used to identify metabolic and environmental risk factors. An assessment of the patient's habitual diet and dietary pattern is used to identify which of these risk factors has a nutritional contributor. When results from the urine analysis are used in combination with a thorough nutrition assessment by a registered dietitian (RD), a comprehensive and individualized nutrition care plan can be developed to address the dietary contributors to stone risk factors.

While it is recommended to tailor nutrition therapy to each patient based on his/her demonstrated risk factors, much as is done in pharmacologic therapy where the medication addresses a measured aberration, there are a few guidelines that all stone formers may follow, regardless of the type of stones they form and of their individual risk factors. This chapter provides the rationale for and strategies to implement these recommendations.

M. Wertheim, MS, RD (✉)
Department of Urology, University of Wisconsin Madison,
3253 Medical Foundation Centennial Building, 1685 Highland Avenue,
Madison, WI 53705, USA
e-mail: wertheim@urology.wisc.edu

Energy

Obesity is associated with higher risk for kidney stones through multiple mechanisms. Obese patients tend to have higher urinary excretion of oxalate and uric acid [1], and lower urinary citrate [2]. Obesity is also associated with increased sodium and phosphorus excretion, and urinary pH is inversely associated with body weight. Insulin resistance, frequently seen in obese patients, has also been associated with defects in renal ammonia production, while hyperinsulinemia is reported to increase urinary calcium excretion [1].

Because obesity plays an important role in metabolic stone disease, assessment of a patient's BMI and consideration of the effect of weight on stone risk factors is a part of the nutrition assessment. BMI is calculated either through the use of BMI charts or using the following equation: BMI = (weight in kg)/(height in m^2). A patient with a BMI of 25.0 or greater is overweight, while a patient with a BMI of 30.0 or higher is classified as obese.

Overweight and obese patients should be counseled that weight loss is an important goal for reducing stone risk factors. It is helpful to provide patients with an estimate of their daily calorie needs to promote either energy balance or weight loss. There are multiple equations used to predict energy expenditure. While the Harris–Benedict equation is still used in clinical practice, recent data suggest that the most accurate equations for calculating resting metabolic rate (RMR) are the Mifflin St. Jeor and Livingston equations. These equations are seen below with W = weight (kg), H = height (cm), A = age (years) [3]. RMR is then multiplied by one of the activity factors below (Table 2.1) to determine total energy expenditure.

- *Mifflin St. Jeor*

    Women: RMR = 10W + 6.25H − 5A − 161

    Men: RMR = 10W + 6.25H − 5A + 5

- *Livingston*

    Women: RMR = 248 × W^0.43356 − 5.09A

    Men: RMR = 293 × W^0.4330 − 5.92A

2. General Nutrition Guidelines for All Stone Formers 11

TABLE 2.1. Activity factors for calculating total energy expenditure.

Activity level	Activity factor
Very light activity	1.3
Light activity	1.5
Moderate activity	1.6
Heavy activity	1.9

Fluids

Stone formers may have lower 24-h urine volumes than healthy controls, and increasing fluid intake in patients with a history of stones will decrease stone risk. Increasing fluid intake decreases the concentration of calcium, oxalate, phosphorus, and uric acid in the urine and decreases relative supersaturation of calcium oxalate, brushite, and uric acid [4].

Fluid needs vary between individuals. The daily fluid intake goal needs to be individualized based on a target urine output of at least 2.5 L daily. Extra-renal losses from perspiration, respiration, and stool vary considerably between individuals based on comorbidities, perspiration, occupation, climate, and activity level [5]. Provider considerations in developing individualized daily fluid intake goals include:

1. Patients with chronic loose stools or diarrhea will have increased extra-renal losses that need to be compensated for with increased fluid intake.
2. Patients with occupations or activities that require time outside in the heat with increased sweat losses will require increased fluid intake to compensate.
3. Urinary incontinence, frequent nocturia, occupations with lack of access to restroom for extended periods of time (such as truck drivers, airline pilots, and elementary school teachers) may need a personalized fluid schedule.

Patient strategies in complying with daily fluid intake goals include:

1. Divide the day into 2–3 sections and consume a target volume of fluids in each section. For example, instruct the patient to consume 1 L fluids in each of three 5-hour

sections of the day—e.g., from 7 a.m. to 12 p.m., 12 p.m. to 5 p.m., 5 p.m. to 10 p.m.
2. Translate liters to ounces, quarts, or any other volume equivalent that makes sense to each patient.
3. Emphasize low-calorie or no-calorie, low sugar beverages. Also encourage diversity. If patients don't like to drink water, recommend tea, sparkling flavored waters, or water with lemon or a small amount of 100 % fruit juice, or low sodium vegetable juice.
4. Ask patients to carry a water bottle with either visible volume markings or a container of known volume, such as 1 L (approximately 32-oz.) container. The patient can then be instructed to fill and drink the contents of the bottle three or more times daily.
5. Adjust fluid intake schedules as needed to accommodate patients' concerns. For nocturia, concentrating fluid intake earlier in the day is helpful. For urinary incontinence, higher fluid intake should be at times when the patient is at home or otherwise has access to facilities.

Sodium

The average sodium intake of Americans is estimated to be about 3,000 mg/day or about double the Dietary Reference Intake of 1,500 mg for ages 9–50. After age 50 and up to age 70, daily sodium requirement is 1,300 mg and lowers further after age 70–1,200 mg. High dietary sodium intake can increase urinary calcium excretion, thus increasing the potential for the formation of calcium-containing stones such as calcium oxalate stones. Sodium expands the extracellular volume and competes with calcium ions for reabsorption in the renal tubule. High sodium intake thus leads to increased sodium being reabsorbed in the renal tubule, leading to increased excretion of calcium [5]. High sodium intake has been shown to lead to increased risk of cystine stones and greater urinary saturation of brushite and monosodium urate. High sodium intake also has the ability to decrease urinary excretion of citrate, an inhibitor of calcium oxalate stone formation [6].

About 75 % of salt intake in the US comes from salt added during processing or manufacturing, not salt added at the table or during cooking. Foods with high sodium content include processed and packaged foods such as deli meats, frozen and canned meals, and certain condiments (e.g., soy sauce). Many people eat bread multiple times daily, and with 200–300 mg sodium per slice, bread is frequently a major source of daily sodium. In contrast, fresh meats, legumes, unprocessed whole grains, fruits, and vegetables are naturally low in sodium. The salt shaker is generally a much smaller contributor to daily sodium intake than processed foods [5]. When buying packaged foods, instruct patients to look for foods that are "sodium free" or "salt free" or "low sodium." Purchasing "reduced sodium" options is helpful but does not guarantee that a food is actually low in sodium. Reduced sodium merely means the food has 25 % less sodium than regular version (Table 2.2).

Citrate

Urinary citrate is an inhibitor of calcium oxalate and phosphate stones through the binding of citrate to calcium to form a soluble complex, leaving calcium unavailable to bind to oxalate or phosphate. Urinary citrate is affected by intake of citrate in the diet, renal acid load, potassium intake, and the presence of frequent diarrhea.

Dietary Citrate

Urinary citrate levels can be altered by dietary intake of citrate. The richest sources of dietary citrate are citrus fruits with lemon and lime being the most concentrated sources. Other citrus fruits have considerably less citrate including oranges, and grapefruit [7, 8]. Strategies for increasing dietary citrate include:

1. Drink 4 oz. lemon or lime juice diluted in water daily. (Note: patients should always be instructed to dilute the juice in order to prevent damage to tooth enamel)

2. Reduce dietary acid load by reducing portions of meat, eggs, and fish, while increasing fruit and vegetable intake
3. Reduce dietary sodium

Renal Acid Load

High dietary acid load may impact urinary citrate levels through enhanced renal reabsorption of citrate. The Potential Renal Acid Load (PRAL) for a particular food takes into account the quantity of chloride, phosphate, sulfate (the acidifying components) and sodium, potassium, calcium, and magnesium (the alkalizing components). Foods that have a positive PRAL include meat, fish, eggs, cheese, grains, and legumes, with animal products generally having a higher dietary acid load per serving than grains or legumes. Dairy products like yogurt and milk are neutral, while fruits and vegetables are generally alkalizing to varying degrees [9].

Minimizing intake of meat and fish, and encouraging intake of fruits and vegetables to five or more servings of fruits and vegetables per day is an important way to help reduce acid load. Tips for increasing fruit and vegetable intake include:

1. Add vegetables like mushrooms, kale, or tomatoes to scrambled eggs or a frittata
2. Add a piece of fruit like berries, apple, or banana to breakfast
3. Snack on clementines or an apple with peanut butter or berries with yogurt, or raw vegetables with hummus
4. Have a big salad for lunch with high-protein vegetables like black or garbanzo beans
5. Keep carrots, celery, or snap peas on hand to add as an easy side dish
6. Reheat frozen vegetables to accompany any meal
7. Sauté mushrooms with garlic and a green vegetable like broccoli or kale
8. Blend up berries or other fruit into a smoothie for a healthy dessert

2. General Nutrition Guidelines for All Stone Formers   15

TABLE 2.2. Foods with high sodium content to limit if intake is excessive.

Cheese	Deli meats and cured meats and fish (such as smoked salmon or lox)	Breakfast meats like sausage and bacon
Frozen meals	Canned soups	Canned vegetables
Chips, pretzels, and other salty snacks	Fast food meals	Canned and jarred tomato sauces and salsas
Some breakfast cereals	Vegetable juices like V8	Casseroles made with canned soups
Breads, bagels, rolls, and baked goods	Hot dogs, bratwurst, sausages, braunschweiger	Pizza and lasagna
Pickles and olives	Some spice blends with added salt	Some salad dressing
Ramen noodles and other dried noodle packets	Boxed meals like macaroni and cheese or hamburger helper, rice-a-roni type meals/sides	

9. Eat spaghetti squash or zucchini noodles as a substitute for pasta
10. Eat butternut squash, sweet potatoes, or carrots as a starch with dinner

Potassium Intake

Urinary potassium excretion is also highly correlated with urinary citrate, and hypokalemia has been established as a cause of hypocitraturia. In hypokalemia, intracellular pH decreases, causing the secretion of hydrogen ions in the kidney resulting in hypocitraturia [10]. Potassium is widely distributed in the food supply with meat, potatoes, fruits, and vegetables all providing varying amounts. Especially good food sources of potassium are potatoes, bananas, tomatoes, oranges, and spinach. High potassium foods also tend to be foods with a lower PRAL, so these foods have the added benefit of reducing overall acid load.

Chronic Diarrhea

Chronic diarrhea can have multiple etiologies including Crohn's disease, ulcerative colitis, short bowel, celiac disease, or other etiologies. Frequent diarrhea results in increased losses of bicarbonate in the stool leading to increased renal absorption of citrate. Managing the underlying cause of the diarrhea is the best way to manage this cause of hypocitraturia. Using dietary or supplemental soluble fiber can help to bulk the stool thus preventing or slowing diarrhea. Good food sources of soluble fiber include apples, pears, bananas, oatmeal, and chia seeds. Probiotic foods and supplements may also be helpful in managing diarrhea [5].

Summary

Body weight, fluid and sodium intake, and urinary citrate levels can all contribute to stone risk in the majority of stone formers. Dietary changes can be effective ways to reduce stone risk factors such as obesity, low urine volume, hyperoxaluria, hypercalciuria, and hypocitraturia. While a thorough assessment of a patient's current diet is essential in order to provide targeted nutrition therapies, the general recommendations provided in this chapter may, without inducing any harm, benefit most all calcium and uric acid stone formers.

References

1. Taylor EN, Stampfer MJ, Curhan GC. Obesity, weight gain, and the risk of kidney stones. JAMA. 2005;294(4):455–62.
2. Asplin JR. Obesity and urolithiasis. Adv Chronic Kidney Dis. 2009;16(1):11–20.
3. Frankenfield DC. Bias and accuracy or resting metabolic rate equations in non-obese and obese adults. Clin Nutr. 2013;32:976–82.
4. Borghi L, Meschi T, Amato F, Briganti A, et al. Urinary volume, water and recurrences in idiopathic calcium nephrolithiasis: a 5-year randomized prospective study. J Urol. 1996;155:839–43.

5. Penniston KL, Nakada SY. Diet and alternative therapies in the management of stone disease. Urol Clin North Am. 2013;40:31–6.
6. Sakhaee K, Harvey J, Padalino P, et al. The potential role of salt abuse on the risk for kidney stone formation. J Urol. 1993;150:310–2.
7. Penniston KL, Steele TH, Nakada SY. Lemonade therapy increases urinary citrate and urine volumes in patients with recurrent calcium oxalate stone formation. J Urol. 2007;70(5):856–60.
8. Seltzer MA, Low RK, McDonald M, et al. Dietary manipulation with lemonade to treat hypocitraturic calcium nephrolithiasis. J Urol. 1996;156:907–9.
9. Remer T. Potential renal acid load of foods and its influence on pH. J Am Diet Assoc. 1995;95(7):791–7.
10. Domrongkitchaiporn S, Stitchantrakul W, Kochakarn W. Causes of hypocitraturia in recurrent calcium stone formers: focusing on urinary potassium excretion. Am J Kidney Dis. 2006;48(4):546–54.

Chapter 3
24-Hour Urine and Serum Tests: When and What?

R. Allan Jhagroo

Serum and 24-Hour Urine Tests: When and What?

Kidney stone disease is common; recurrence can be estimated at 52 % in 10 years [1]. Both blood and urine tests can be helpful for kidney stone prevention. Deciding when and what to order is often not very clear, and indications for such tests may vary by practice preference in addition to patient variables. This chapter will attempt to provide the reasoning used to guide the ordering of lab tests in the work up of kidney stone disease. As patients are unique, a clinical impression may provide the primary rationale for ordering certain tests. The clinical opinion of the author is expressed in much of this chapter as evidence is insufficient for much of this topic.

R.A. Jhagroo, MD (✉)
Department of Medicine and Urology, University of Wisconsin Madison, 3034 Fish Hatchery Road, Madison, WI 53713, USA
e-mail: rajhagroo@medicine.wisc.edu

Who Should Get Further Testing After Forming a Kidney Stone?

Primary prevention of kidney stones with conservative measures such as increasing fluid intake may be financially beneficial if applied broadly [2]. However, it may be unreasonable to expect changes at the population level without the motivation of a previous stone event. Currently, tests of patients' blood and urine are offered to patients with multiple stones, recurrent stones, bilateral stones, unique stones, stones large in size, and in stone formers of young age. More simply, a history of anything in addition to a single moderately sized kidney stone warrants further evaluation. Occasionally, some single stone formers receive blood and urine evaluations in order to prevent future kidney stones. With emerging data to support the association of stones with systemic diseases, such as cardiovascular [3] and premature bone loss [4], the urgency of kidney stone management may be changing. At this time, selection of who should receive these tests remains individualized, as testing all patients remains controversial.

Evaluation and management for the patient who has formed a single kidney stone requires justification. It is important to keep in mind that the prevention of kidney stones requires significant patient effort. In the instance of diet, patients may be asked to make changes to their eating habits for the rest of their lives. If a medication is prescribed, it is important for patients to recognize that its use is often not temporary. Typically, medications work best in conjunction with diet changes. A good example is the use of thiazide-type medications for the treatment of hypercalciuria. In this example, if sodium restriction is not practiced the medication's positive effect may be dampened and potassium losses magnified. For this reason, the screening of patients to elicit willingness to make changes in diet or to take medications is useful. The effort required to collect a 24-h urine sample requires some level of motivation and may predict the willingness to make preventive changes. Most patients may not be able to commit to being willing to make diet changes or take medications unless results of testing demonstrate risk of recurrence. For those who openly state they are not interested in medications or diet manipulations, further testing may not be useful. At that point, education regarding risk of future stones and general recommendations may be given, and patients can undergo testing in the future if interest changes.

What Tests Should Be Ordered?

It has been suggested that ordering all tests on all patients is not the best approach from a cost perspective [5]. However, specific blood and urine tests may lead to correction of underlying conditions predisposing to kidney stones, such as hyperparathyroidism or sarcoidosis. For this reason, determining which tests should be ordered on which patients is critical.

Basic Blood Chemistry

A basic metabolic panel (BMP) including serum bicarbonate and calcium is done on the majority of patients who have an acute stone event. A BMP may be missing at the time of evaluation and should subsequently be obtained on every stone former regardless of interest in making lifestyle changes. At least one BMP should be obtained at a time when acute illness is not present and in conjunction with a 24-h urine test. Further details regarding the utility of blood tests are shown in Table 3.1.

Serum Calcium and Hyperparathyroidism

Hyperparathyroidism is reported to be present in 2–8 % of kidney stone formers [6]. Therefore, those seen in a stone clinic or stone referral center have a higher likelihood of having this glandular disorder, and the degree of suspicion for hyperparathyroidism should be relatively high.

Table 3.1 Specific serum lab tests and their utility.

Test	Utility
BMP (basic metabolic panel)	Should include calcium, potassium, bicarbonate, creatinine, sodium and glucose
Serum calcium total/ionized	High in hyperparathyroidism. May be more sensitive while the patient is under the treatment of thiazide-like medications. The upper limit of normal should still be considered high if PTH is not suppressed. Assessment of ionized calcium may help when total calcium is not clearly elevated
Serum glucose	May serve as indicator for further testing to pursue a diagnosis of diabetes, which is associated with lower urine pH and uric acid stones
Serum bicarbonate	May serve as an indicator of systemic acidosis, which is associated with increased stone risk, especially in the setting of a distal RTA
Serum potassium	High levels would prompt follow-up labs if potassium citrate is prescribed, especially if additional hyperkalemia-causing medications are concomitantly prescribed or if chronic kidney disease exists. Low levels would prohibit use of thiazide-like medications until corrected, and will need to be followed closely if prescribed
Serum sodium	Low sodium would prohibit the use of thiazide-type medications
Parathyroid axis (PTH, calcium, 25-OH vitamin D, phosphorus)	Evaluated if serum calcium is >10.0 mg/dL OR if calcium phosphate stones OR if high urine pH and calcium
PTH	Serves as marker of the level of activity of the parathyroid gland. Should be done at the same time as the rest of the PTH axis
Phosphorus	May be low with high 24-h urine excretion in the setting of hyperparathyroidism. Rarely, may represent a primary renal phosphate leak
25-OH vitamin D	Can be useful to completely define findings from the PTH axis as low vitamin D, in association with elevated PTH, may suggest secondary hyperparathyroidism. Also useful to rule out vitamin D intoxication
Additional tests below	
Magnesium	Magnesium replacement is indicated if hypomagnesemia is detected, especially in patients with hypokalemia
Uric acid	Occasionally useful to guide therapy of calcium stones with xanthine oxidase inhibitors in patients with hyperuricosuria. Useful to follow in patients with gout on thiazide medications
1,25 vitamin D	Only if sarcoid, other granulomatous diseases, or malignancies are suspected

Serum calcium evaluation is the simplest way to screen for hyperparathyroidism, but it may not be persistently elevated, and defining the upper limit of abnormal has been difficult. A blatantly high serum calcium (>10.5 mg/dL on most total calcium assays) may prompt immediate testing and diagnosis of hyperparathyroidism. Surgical treatment by removal of the gland(s) may then correct the problem. But serum calcium within normal laboratory ranges should not necessarily rule out further work up. Normal calcium in hyperparathyroidism has been described and is not rare in stone formers. The fact that the patient has already formed a stone should heighten suspicion of abnormal parathyroid activity, and normal serum calcium in this case should not end the evaluation for it.

The Parathyroid Axis

If calcium phosphate is present in at least 5 % of a patient's stone, the parathyroid axis (blood calcium, phosphorus, parathyroid hormone, and 25-OH vitamin D) should be tested, even if serum calcium was previously normal. To evaluate for phosphorus and calcium wasting, fractional excretion of phosphorus and calcium can be checked when the blood tests are being done. These tests may identify patients with elevated urine phosphorus, low serum phosphorus, and relatively normal PTH levels, which would suggest a primary leak of phosphorus at the level of the kidney. A check of 1,25 vitamin D is not needed in the majority of patients. However, if sarcoidosis or malignancy is suspected, this test should be done. Hypophosphatemia may suggest disorders of renal phosphate reabsorption such as mutations in the genes encoding the sodium-phosphate cotransporters.

All patients with serum calcium >10.0 mg/dL should have blood tests to evaluate the parathyroid axis as well as 24-h urine stone risk assessment. Patients nearing 10.0 mg/dL of total calcium may be found to have even higher calcium values with a test of ionized calcium. If it is not revealing, it may need to be repeated if changes in urine, blood, or stone analyses occur.

24-h Urine Tests

Testing for multiple variables in a 24-h urine collection eliminates the guesswork about potential aberrations and usually also provides information about supersaturation. Several commercial laboratories provide risk "profiles" that provide information from a single 24-h urine collection about both stone promoters and inhibitors. In the single stone former with no radiographic evidence of additional stones, it may not be necessary to order a 24-h urine test. However, age and other comorbidities may justify it. Early intervention after an initial stone event may be most effective in preventing recurrence [7]. While a single 24-h urine test is laborsome, there is a >90 % detection rate [8] of treatable abnormalities when 2–3 studies are completed [9]. With only one study, the impact of collection error can be easily overlooked as predicted creatinine may not identify all inaccurate collections. With a second collection that corroborates collection adequacy, we can be more confident of the evaluation. If the 24-h urinary creatinine values differ by more than 30 %, a third collection can help isolate the more accurate studies. As many patients have the 24-h urine test done shortly after stone formation, diet changes may have been made, and the test may not therefore reveal the risk factors present when the stone was formed. For this reason, a second or third test 6–12 months after the stone event may be better reflective of the patient's typical diet. In the instance of only one test being available, diet modifications may be made until confirmatory 24-h urine results are available to support the use of prescription medications.

While lab tests are helpful in ruling out causative diseases such as hyperparathyroidism, they are only a part of the clinical picture. Management should incorporate other factors such as stone burden, frequency, and type, patient age, and comorbidities. Figure 3.1 provides an overview of patient evaluation.

3. 24-Hour Urine and Serum Tests: When and What?

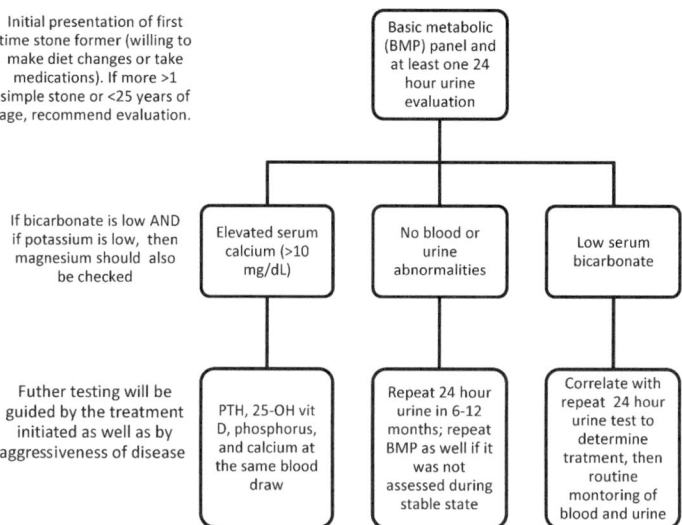

Fig. 3.1. Guidance for targeting the groups of patients that would most benefit from the particular laboratory test.

Am I Missing Something?

In the case of particular diagnoses that are less common, it is important to know when to look further. In addition to hyperparathyroidism and renal tubular acidosis, which are readily treatable, other underlying causes of stones exist. For the most part, younger age in the patient with stones triggers a closer look for underlying disease. Cystine stone formers are typically identified with stone analysis, although the urologist often is aware of the diagnosis based on the physical features of the stone at the time of treatment. Management of cystine stones is significantly different from that of calcium-based stones; cystinuria should therefore be identified for that reason. Cystine screening is a routine part of many but not all 24-h urine evaluations that are geared to kidney stone prevention, but it can also be detected on microscopy or via specifically ordered testing. Genetic diseases presenting at younger ages with multiple stones, such as primary hyperoxaluria, Lowe's, and Dent's disease, have other characteristic findings that accompany them.

References

1. Uribarri J, Oh MS, Carroll HJ. The first kidney stone. Ann Intern Med. 1989;111(12):1006–9. Epub 1989/12/15.
2. Lotan Y, Buendia Jimenez I, Lenoir-Wijnkoop I, Daudon M, Molinier L, Tack I, et al. Primary prevention of nephrolithiasis is cost-effective for a national healthcare system. BJU Int. 2012;110(11 Pt C):E1060–7. Epub 2012/06/13.
3. Rule AD, Roger VL, Melton 3rd LJ, Bergstralh EJ, Li X, Peyser PA, et al. Kidney stones associate with increased risk for myocardial infarction. J Am Soc Nephrol. 2010;21(10):1641–4. Epub 2010/07/10.
4. Melton 3rd LJ, Crowson CS, Khosla S, Wilson DM, O'Fallon WM. Fracture risk among patients with urolithiasis: a population-based cohort study. Kidney Int. 1998;53(2):459–64. Epub 1998/02/14.
5. Chandhoke PS. When is medical prophylaxis cost-effective for recurrent calcium stones? J Urol. 2002;168(3):937–40. Epub 2002/08/21.
6. Rodman JS, Mahler RJ. Kidney stones as a manifestation of hypercalcemic disorders. Hyperparathyroidism and sarcoidosis. Urol Clin North Am. 2000;27(2):275–85, viii. Epub 2000/04/25.
7. Parks JH, Coe FL. An increasing number of calcium oxalate stone events worsens treatment outcome. Kidney Int. 1994;45(6):1722–30. Epub 1994/06/01.
8. Hess B, Hasler-Strub U, Ackermann D, Jaeger P. Metabolic evaluation of patients with recurrent idiopathic calcium nephrolithiasis. Nephrol Dial Transplant. 1997;12(7):1362–8. Epub 1997/07/01.
9. Parks JH, Goldfisher E, Asplin JR, Coe FL. A single 24-hour urine collection is inadequate for the medical evaluation of nephrolithiasis. J Urol. 2002;167(4):1607–12. Epub 2002/03/26.

Part II
Calcium Stones

Chapter 4
Nutrition Management of Hypercalciuria

E. Susannah Southern

Dietary Calcium

Reducing dietary intake of calcium has historically been targeted as a means of managing hypercalciuria. Recommendations for dietary calcium restriction were common for patients with hypercalciuria and for calcium stone formers. Although higher dietary calcium intake can increase intestinal absorption of calcium and subsequently increase urinary calcium excretion, calcium restriction does not appear to reduce the risk of stone formation. Large observational studies have, in fact, shown a significant *inverse* relationship between dietary calcium intake and risk of kidney stones, with a 34 % increased risk in young men with low calcium intake and similar results for young women and older women [1]. This may be due to a resultant increase of free oxalate absorption from the intestine with a low intake of oxalate-binding calcium. Additionally, dairy products, the primary source of

---

E.S. Southern, RDN, LDN (✉)
Department of Nutrition & Food Services, UNC Health Care,
UNC Outpatient Nutrition Clinic, Aycock Family Medicine,
590 Manning Drive, Chapel Hill, NC 27599-7586, USA
e-mail: Susannah.southern@unchealthcare.unc.edu

dietary calcium, may offer protection against kidney stones related to other inhibitory factors of nephrolithiasis such as dietary potassium.

Patients with idiopathic hypercalciuria do not see reductions in urinary calcium excretion equal to the reduction in calcium ingested when placed on a restricted calcium diet [2]. This suggests an increase in bone resorption of calcium. Therefore, finding other ways to reduce urinary calcium concentration is warranted for protection of bone density as well as for stone prevention. Calcium supplementation has been observed to increase urinary calcium excretion, though the effect varies related to timing and dosage. For example, calcium supplements ingested without food and thus in the absence of its potential intestinal binders, such as oxalate and phytate, lead to greater intestinal calcium absorption and urinary excretion than when supplements are consumed at meals [1].

In light of the lack of evidence for stone prevention through calcium restriction and the risk of bone demineralization, the consensus recommendation for stone prevention is a moderate intake of dietary calcium consistent with the Dietary Reference Intakes for life stage and gender groups (1,000–1,300 mg for individuals from 9 years old through adulthood or approximately 3–4 servings of calcium-rich foods per day). If calcium supplements are needed to reach total intake recommendations, they should be taken with or shortly after meals and only in the dosage required to bring total calcium intake to goal.

Dietary Sodium

Dietary sodium is a contributor to hypercalciuria related to sodium's expansion of extracellular volume and sodium ion competition with calcium in the renal tubule. There is a 25–40 mg increase in urinary calcium for every 100 mEq increase (2,300 mg or the amount in one teaspoon or packet of salt) in dietary sodium intake per day [3]. Excretion of urinary calcium has been demonstrated to vary directly with changes in dietary sodium in kidney stone-forming patients [4]. In addition, lower bone density has been observed in stone formers with high sodium diets [5]. It is therefore worthwhile to advise these patients to reduce their intake of dietary sodium if it is high and if it is thought to contribute to excessive calciuria.

Recommendations to lower sodium intake are based ideally on an assessment that identifies a patient's highest sodium contributors as well as those foods that contribute significantly to total sodium intake due to frequent consumption [6]. The American Heart Association targets bread as the top dietary contributor to American sodium intake. This is mainly due to the high frequency of bread intake in the typical American diet rather than the moderate sodium content of most bread servings.

Reducing sodium intake to 1,500–2,300 mg per day is desirable. This range is the recommendation from the 2010 Dietary Guidelines for Americans, the upper value being the daily sodium recommendation for healthy young adults and the lower being the target for those over age 50, African Americans, those with hypertension or with other risk factors [7].

Medical nutrition therapy provided by a registered dietitian nutritionist is valuable for guiding patients who need dietary sodium reduction for better stone prevention. Many patients will claim that they do not eat a lot of salt, but dietary assessment can help them understand their sodium intake beyond the salt shaker.

Acid Load of the Diet

A high dietary acid load contributes to hypercalciuria by decreasing renal tubular calcium reabsorption, increasing calcium bone resorption to buffer the acid load, increasing glomerular filtration rate, and/or increasing calcium absorption in the intestine [8]. Therefore, for patients with hypercalciuria, it is helpful to assess dietary intake of the types of foods that raise the acid load of the diet and recommended changes if needed [9]. The Potential Renal Acid Load (PRAL) of foods has been estimated and a scale developed. Foods with a high PRAL are:

- Foods of flesh origin from both land and water
- Cheeses (mainly hard cheeses), eggs (mainly from the yolk)
- Grains, nearly all types when consumed frequently and/or in large quantities

Foods that confer an alkaline load include nearly all fruits and vegetables. A few, such as cranberries and lentils, have a slight acid load, but not enough to restrict them from the diet. This is an important distinction as fruits and vegetables are nearly always encouraged for their stone prevention properties. Milk, yogurt, and fats are neutral and do not affect the acid load of the diet. Manipulation of the acid load of the diet by shifting some flesh protein sources to more neutral or alkalinizing protein choices, by increasing intake of fruits and vegetables, and by moderating intake of grain foods may effectively reduce urinary calcium excretion.

Other Dietary Factors

Fiber

Intake of dietary fiber is worth assessing for adequacy as fiber may be able to reduce gastrointestinal absorption of calcium [9]. This would be warranted in those with normal bone and calcium status who also need reduction in urinary calcium. Getting daily fiber intake up to the normal recommended level of 25–30 g per day by advising patients to choose whole grains over refined as well as having adequate intake of whole fruits, vegetables, and legumes would be appropriate. The phytate and oxalate content of these foods may also play a role in their ability to reduce calcium absorption.

Carbohydrates

Intake of a high carbohydrate diet may transiently increase urinary calcium excretion [9]. Advising patients with a high intake of refined carbohydrates (sweetened drinks, juices, processed grains, sweets, and foods with significant added sugar such as sugary breakfast cereals) to choose less refined whole grains, whole fruits, and low calorie beverages may reduce urinary calcium.

Weight Loss

Boosting fiber intake and limiting refined carbohydrate consumption are also good recommendations for patients attempting weight loss for reduction of stone risk. These patients would likely experience greater satiety from the fiber bulk and would reduce caloric intake via a reduction of less satiating calories from liquids and processed carbohydrates.

Alcohol and Caffeine

Intake of alcohol and caffeine has also been linked to increases in urinary calcium excretion [9]. Assessment of individual intake and recommendations for moderation, if indicated, may reduce stone risk.

Fish Oil

The possible role in urological health for omega-3 fatty acids from fish oil is under investigation. It has been observed that Greenland Eskimos, who have a dietary pattern high in omega-3 fatty acids from fish, have a low incidence of nephrolithiasis [10], presumably from lower urinary calcium excretion. One proposed mechanism for omega-3 fatty acid intake and reduced calciuria relates to changes in prostaglandin production due to a higher ratio of omega-3 to omega-6 fatty acids. Arachadonic acid (AA), a non-essential fatty acid and the most commonly consumed omega-6 fatty acid, is the precursor of prostaglandin E2 (PGE2), a pro-inflammatory lipid mediator. High levels of PGE2 are correlated with high urinary calcium excretion. In contrast, eicosapentaenoic acid (EPA), an omega-3 fatty acid, is a required nutrient for humans and is found in fish. It competes with AA for cyclooxygenase and lowers production of AA metabolites, including PGE2. Studies have shown increased urinary calcium excretion with a dietary intake high in AA and low in EPA [10]. PGE2 also stimulates the rate of bone resorption as it increases the production of calcitriol, the active form of vitamin D. Thus, an increase in the omega-3, omega-6 intake ratio is another potential mechanism for reduced hypercalciuria and nephrolithiasis. Finally, incorporation of EPA in cell membranes at the expense of AA may protect from lipid peroxidation and the cell membrane injury that can lead to stone development.

Summary

Evidence suggests that dietary modifications can reduce urinary calcium excretion and prevent the formation of new stones. To summarize:

- Consume adequate dietary calcium of 1,000–1,200 mg per day from three to four servings of dairy or non-dairy calcium containing foods.
- If needed to meet daily calcium intake guidelines, take up to 300 mg of calcium citrate as a supplement with a meal.
- Limit daily sodium intake to 1,500–2,300 mg per day by avoiding foods that are very high in sodium and by modifying intake frequency of the top total dietary sodium contributors such as bread, luncheon meats, and cheese.
- Reduce the acid load of the diet by balancing intake of foods that confer a high acid load—such as fleshy proteins (all meats, poultry, fish, seafood), cheeses, egg yolks,

and large quantities of grains—with more neutral or alkalinizing choices such as fruits, vegetables, milk, yogurt, and healthy fats.
- Consume adequate dietary fiber of 25–30 g per day from fruits, vegetables, legumes, and whole grains.
- Moderate intake of refined carbohydrates from sugar sweetened drinks, juices, and processed carbohydrates and desserts.
- Moderate intake of alcohol and caffeine if high intake is present.
- Consider taking an omega 3 supplement from fish oil (specific dosages to reduce calciuria are not know, but 2,000–3,000 mg fish oil daily is an estimated safe target).

References

1. Heilberg IP, Goldfarb DS. Nutrition and chronic kidney disease optimum nutrition for kidney stone disease clinical summary. Adv Chronic Kidney Dis. 2013;20(2):165–74.
2. Coe FL, Favus MJ, Crockett T, et al. Effects of low-calcium diet on urine calcium excretion, parathyroid function and serum 1, 25(OH)2D3 levels in patients with idiopathic hypercalciuria and in normal subjects. Am J Med. 1982;72:25–32.
3. Bleich HL, Moore MJ, Lemann J, et al. Urinary calcium excretion in human beings. N Engl J Med. 1979;301:535–41.
4. Muldowney FP, Freaney R, Moloney MF, et al. Importance of dietary sodium in the hypercalciuria syndrome. Kidney Int. 1982;22:292–6.
5. Martini LA, Cuppari L, Colugnati FA, et al. High sodium chloride intake is associated with low bone density in calcium stone-forming patients. Clin Nephrol. 2000;54:85–93.
6. Penniston KL, Wojciechowski KF, Nakada SY. The salt shaker provides less than 15 % of the total sodium intake in stone formers: food strategies to reduce sodium are needed. J Urol. 2011;185:e861.
7. United States Department of Agriculture. Department of Health and Human Services. Dietary Guidelines for Americans; 2010. http://health.gov/dietaryguidelines/dga2010/dietaryguidelines2010.pdf. Accessed 12 Jan 2014.

8. Remer T. Influence of diet on acid–base balance. Semin Dial. 2000;13(4):221–6.
9. Penniston KL, Nakada SY. Diet and alternative therapies in the management of stone disease. Urol Clin North Am. 2013; 40:31–46.
10. Ortiz-Alvarado O, Miyaoka R, Kreidberg C, Leavitt DA, Moeding A, Stessman M, Monga M. Omega-3 fatty acids eicosapentaenoic acid and docosahexaenoic acid in the management of hypercalciuric stone formers. Urology. 2012;79(2):282–6.

Chapter 5
Medical Management of Hypercalciuria

Sushant R. Taksande and Anna L. Zisman

Introduction

Nearly 80 % patients with nephrolithiasis have calcium-based stones. Hypercalciuria is the most common metabolic abnormality in calcium stone formers, with about 50 % of patients with stone disease demonstrating the trait. It may be defined as >250 mg/day of urine calcium in females and >300 mg/day in males. However, the risk of stones increases as urine calcium excretion increases even at values below these thresholds, suggesting that urine calcium should be considered a linear function, rather than a binary "normal" vs. "high." Increasing urine calcium concentration alters the urinary supersaturation of calcium oxalate and calcium phosphate and is thus directly linked to increased risk of calcium stone disease [1].

Etiology

The most common etiology of hypercalciuria is genetic hypercalciuria, often termed idiopathic hypercalciuria. Approximately 50 % of first degree relatives of a patient with hypercalciuria without an apparent systemic cause will also demonstrate hypercalciuria, suggesting an autosomal dominant pattern of inheritance, though the trait appears to be polygenic. A careful history and a high index of suspicion may help guide further evaluation or will help eliminate secondary causes of increased urinary calcium excretion including:

Primary hyperparathyroidism—a normal serum calcium generally excludes this diagnosis, but a high index of suspicion is necessary for subtle cases.
Vitamin D excess—exogenous vitamin D, granulomatous disease (sarcoidosis, lymphoma, tuberculosis).
Hyperthyroidism—it is also important to make sure that in the setting of thyroid replacement therapy, the doses remain appropriate over time.
Renal Tubular Acidosis—the diagnosis is suggested by a low serum bicarbonate concentration.
Vitamin A toxicity
Medication use

Corticosteroids, acetazolamide, topiramate

Immobility
Paget's disease
Genetic/congenital abnormalities [2]

Calcium sensing receptor (CaSR) mutations
Dent's disease (chloride channel 5 mutations)
Bartter's syndrome (mutations in multiple genes affecting ion transport in the ascending limb of the loop of Henle)
Liddle's syndrome (ENaC mutations)
Hereditary hypophosphatemic rickets with hypercalciuria
Medullary sponge kidney
Beckwith—Weidmann syndrome
Familial hypomagnesemia (claudin 16, claudin 19 mutations)
Osteogenesis imperfecta type 1

Diagnosis

The diagnosis of hypercalciuria is established with at least one 24-h urine collection demonstrating excess calcium excretion [1] as defined by at least one of the following:

- An absolute value of greater than 250 mg of calcium per day in females or >300 mg of calcium per day in males. Even values significantly below these "thresholds" however may be worth lowering in patients with recurrent stones.
- Urinary calcium excretion of greater than 4 mg/kg of body weight.
- Urinary calcium excretion of greater than 140 mg/g creatinine.

Definitions based on factoring calcium excretion for body weight or creatinine excretion may be useful in children and older people or others with reduced muscle mass.

Complications

In addition to risk of stone disease, hypercalciuria carries with it a risk of bone demineralization and osteoporosis [3].

- Hypercalciuric patients often excrete more calcium than they absorb leading to a negative calcium balance and bone loss.
- Bone mineral density is inversely correlated with degree of hypercalciuria in both male and female hypercalciuric stone formers (but not non-stone formers).
- Stone formers have a higher incidence of both vertebral and long bone fracture compared to non-stone formers in multiple epidemiological studies.
- Consider performing Dual Emission X-ray Absorptiometry (DEXA) in patients with hypercalciuria, particularly post-menopausal women and either gender with a family history of osteoporosis or bone fracture.

Treatment

General Considerations

Hypercalciuria portends a risk of kidney stone formation. General kidney stone prevention guidelines apply to patients with hypercalciuria including

- High fluid intake to yield at least 2–2.5 L of urine volume.
- Sodium restricted diet of less than 2,000–2,300 mg per day.
- Moderation of animal protein intake to 0.8–1 g/kg per day.
- Avoidance of calcium supplements and age-appropriate intake of dietary calcium (1,000 mg of elemental calcium between the ages of 19 and 50, 1,200 mg in patients older than 50 years).

Pharmacological Treatment of Hypercalciuria

Treatment of hypercalciuria to decrease supersaturation for calcium oxalate and calcium phosphate decreases the risk of recurrent nephrolithiasis. Given the linear nature of urine calcium excretion, applying these therapies only to patients meeting the threshold definitions of hypercalciuria discussed above may be too restrictive and will preclude giving effective therapy to all those who may benefit. As discussed below, thiazides have been shown to prevent stones even in patients who do not meet these threshold definitions of hypercalciuria.

General Indications for Pharmacological Treatment

- Clinical or radiological evaluation showing worsening stone disease on conservative treatment after first episode of symptomatic stone and evidence of hypercalciuria on metabolic evaluation.
- Multiple stones detected on imaging with evidence of hypercalciuria with or without clinical symptoms.

- Can be strongly considered in first time stone former with evidence of higher magnitudes of hypercalciuria on metabolic evaluation.
- Osteopenia or osteoporosis.

Pharmacotherapy

Thiazide Diuretics

Mechanism of Action

- Thiazides block sodium reabsorption in distal convoluted tubule leading to natriuresis, mild extracellular volume depletion, and a consequent upregulation of calcium absorption in proximal tubule. In addition there might be a component of direct enhancement of calcium absorption in the distal nephron.
- Thiazides cause increased excretion of certain inhibitors of crystallization like magnesium, zinc, and pyrophosphate. In addition, long-term use may reduce urine oxalate levels.

Efficacy

1. Reducing Hypercalciuria:
   - In experimental studies, indapamide and hydrochlorothiazide (HCTZ) were shown to result in up to 50 % reduction in 24-h calcium levels in patients with idiopathic hypercalciuria [4, 5].
   - Indapamide caused a 48 % reduction in 24-h calciuria in a larger clinical trial.
2. Reducing Stone recurrence:
   - Current evidence indicates that HCTZ in doses of 50 mg/day [6], chlorthalidone 25–50 mg/day, and indapamide 2.5 mg/day are effective in reducing stone recurrences in patients with or without hypercalciuria at baseline [7].

Individual Medications

1. Hydrochlorthiazide

   - Starting dose may be 25 mg but goal dose for treatment with HCTZ is 50 mg/day or 25 mg bid. Note that it is higher than doses used commonly for treatment of hypertension.
   - The hypocalciuric effect of HCTZ is dose dependent. Though doses up to 200 mg/day have been used in the clinical trials, these are limited by metabolic abnormalities associated with thiazides like hypokalemia, hypomagnesemia, and metabolic alkalosis.
   - HCTZ is also available as a combination tablet with amiloride: 50 mg HCTZ with 5 mg amiloride. An effective dose is often ½ tablet twice a day.

2. Chlorthalidone

   - Chlorthalidone has significantly longer half-life allowing for once daily dosing. It can be used in doses of 25–50 mg/day and is equivalent in hypocalciuric efficacy to HCTZ.
   - May have greater hypokalemic effect than HCTZ and require increased potassium supplementation.

3. Indapamide

   - Indapamide is typically used in doses of 2.5 mg per day. Limited data from smaller studies have shown a trend towards better metabolic profile (less hyperuricemia, hypokalemia) and lesser effect on urine citrate reduction than HCTZ.

Adverse Effects

Well-recognized dose dependent adverse effects include metabolic abnormalities such as hypokalemia, mild increases in blood glucose, hyperlipidemia, hyperuricemia, and hypomagnesemia. Mild increases in serum calcium have also been noted. By causing potassium depletion, thiazides cause a reduction in urine citrate levels, and thus the effect on supersaturation of calcium salts may not parallel the hypocalciuric effect [8]. Supplementation with potassium citrate therefore is usually recommended, as citrate excretion is corrected, and hyperglycemia may be prevented. Even potassium chloride supplementation will help maintain citrate excretion. The systemic blood pressure lowering is generally a welcome effect, but can be dose limiting in the healthy young person.

Alkali Therapy in Hypercalciuria

Mechanism of Action

- An alkali load reliably increases urine pH by increasing excretion of the bicarbonate ion. Citrate is converted to bicarbonate by the liver and ultimately the increased serum bicarbonate concentration decreases reabsorption of citrate by the proximal tubule.
- An alkali load may also have an independent mechanism in lowering urine calcium excretion by lowering bone turnover.

Individual Medications

Potassium Citrate

Use

Potassium citrate should be used in situations where thiazide treatment is compounded by hypokalemia or if hypocitraturia is also present. Patients with concurrent hypocitraturia with hypercalciuria should be started on combined therapy at the beginning of treatment.

The initial dose of potassium citrate can be 10 meq 2 or 3 times a day with up to 60 meq/day. Dose can be titrated based on serum potassium concentration and urine pH. Doses up to 100 meq may be required in certain situations particularly with high doses of thiazides, or resistant hypokalemia.

Sodium Potassium Citrate

While the alkali loading effect of a mixed sodium/potassium citrate is similar, the sodium load may blunt the beneficial antilithogenic response of therapy.

Potassium Magnesium Citrate

Potassium magnesium citrate has been shown to be effective in decreasing the rate of calcium oxalate stone formation, as well as in the treatment of thiazide-induced hypokalemia, hypocitraturia, and concomitant hypomagnesemia. Trial data suggest an initial dose equivalent to 14 meq of potassium, 6 meq of magnesium, and 18 meq of citrate three times daily.

Adverse Effects

Gastrointestinal upset is common. If urine pH>6.5, potentially increased risk for calcium phosphate stone formation may result. However, the effect of citrate to inhibit calcium stone formation makes this a rare event.

Neutral Phosphates

Mechanism of Action

Neutral phosphates can lower the calcitriol levels and reduce absorption of calcium from the gut, reducing urinary calcium excretion. Levels of urinary pyrophosphate, an inhibitor of calcium crystallization may also increase with therapy.

Efficacy

Potassium phosphate (elemental phosphate of about 600 mg) in divided doses can cause a 30–35 % sustainable reduction in 24 h urine calcium. While no long-term clinical trial data on preventing stone recurrence exist, neutral phosphates can be considered as an alternative in case of thiazide ineffectiveness or intolerance, or in particularly recalcitrant cases. It is used infrequently.

Adverse Effects

Gastrointestinal symptoms limit widespread use.

Amiloride

Amiloride augments the hypocalciuric effect of thiazides [9] though there are no long-term data on stone recurrence rates. Combination therapy with thiazide may limit the hypokalemic and hypocitraturia effects of thiazides. Use of amiloride can also be considered in situations where clinical situation dictates the need for further natriuresis.

Management Issues

Duration of Treatment

- Generally treatment for hypercalciuria is lifelong as risks of stone formation and bone loss return to baseline with cessation of therapy. Trials off therapy with measurement of urine calcium excretion might be worthwhile in patients who have effectively reduced their sodium intake.
- If renal function declines during therapy, typically hypercalciuria will abate due to secondary hyperparathyroidism leading to reduced urine calcium excretion. Ongoing treatment can then be reconsidered.

Monitoring

- Periodic monitoring of serum electrolytes, creatinine, and 24-h urinary parameters is necessary to assure stability of both risk factors and the effects of therapy.

A 50 % reduction in urine calcium excretion is desirable but even lesser degrees of reduction are useful, especially when combined with increased urinary volume and citrate excretion. Our practice is to perform a 24-urine collection and a serum panel with creatinine and electrolytes every 12–24 months in all patients.

Bisphosphonates for Hypercalciuria

Mechanism of Action

Reduction of osteoclast resorption of bone may reduce release of calcium and reduce the kidneys' filtered load.

Use

Some data suggest that bisphosphonates are associated with reductions in urine calcium excretion in patients with hypercalciuria and might therefore reduce calcium stone incidence. Convincing evidence that stone formation is prevented is lacking. They may be useful adjuncts to therapy with or without thiazides, when low bone mineral density is present. They may be useful especially if thiazides are not well tolerated.

Individual Medications

Alendronate, risedronate, ibandronate, and zoledronic acid may all be useful and have not been compared for efficacy in reducing urine calcium excretion or preventing stones.

References

1. Worcester EM, Coe FL. Calcium kidney stones. N Engl J Med. 2010;363:954–63.
2. Stechman MJ, Loh NY, Thakker RV. Genetic causes of hypercalciuric nephrolithiasis. Pediatr Nephrol. 2009;24:2321–32.

5. Medical Management of Hypercalciuria 47

3. Krieger NS, Bushinsky DA. The relation between bone and stone formation. Calcif Tissue Int. 2013;93:374–81.
4. Lemieux G. Treatment of idiopathic hypercalciuria with indapamide. CMAJ. 1986;135(2):119–21.
5. Ceylan K, Topal C, Erkoc R, Sayarlioglu H, Can S, Yilmaz Y, et al. Effect of indapamide on urinary calcium excretion in patients with and without urinary stone disease. Ann Pharmacother. 2005;39(6):1034–8.
6. Fernandez-Rodriguez A, Arrabal-Martin M, Garcia-Ruiz MJ, Arrabal-Polo MA, Pichardo-Pichardo S, Zuluaga-Gomez A. The role of thiazides in the prophylaxis of recurrent calcium lithiasis. Actas Urol Esp. 2006;30(3):305–9.
7. Escribano J, Balaguer A, Pagone F, Feliu A, Roque IFM. Pharmacological interventions for preventing complications in idiopathic hypercalciuria. Cochrane Database Syst Rev. 2009;1:CD004754.
8. Nicar MJ, Peterson R, Pak CY. Use of potassium citrate as potassium supplement during thiazide therapy of calcium nephrolithiasis. J Urol. 1984;131(3):430–3.
9. Alon U, Costanzo LS, Chan JC. Additive hypocalciuric effects of amiloride and hydrochlorothiazide in patients treated with calcitriol. Miner Electrolyte Metab. 1984;10(6):379–86.

Chapter 6
Nutrition Management of Hypocitraturia

Liz Weinandy

Low urinary citrate is a known risk factor for calcium nephrolithiasis. Hypocitraturia is most commonly defined as urine citrate lower than 320 milligrams (mg) in a 24-h period. However, ideal concentrations are thought to be around 600 mg per day, which is the average amount excreted by non-stone forming adults. Adequate citrate in the urine decreases stone formation risk by binding to calcium to form a soluble complex. This reduces the risk for crystal nucleation, aggregation, and growth of both calcium oxalate and calcium phosphate stones [1, 2].

It is estimated that 10–35 % of the filtered renal citrate is excreted in the urine. Low urine citrate may be idiopathic or have a known cause. Non-nutritional causes include the use of certain medications, acid–base disorders, and strenuous exercise [1, 3]. Kidney stones attributed to hypocitraturia may be successfully treated with medical nutrition therapy (MNT), but pharmacologic therapy may be needed for very low urine citrate. Known dietary causes include: high dietary acid load, low carbohydrate diets, low potassium intake, conditions causing diarrhea and malabsorption, low magnesium

---

L. Weinandy, MPH, RD, LD (✉)
Nutrition Services, Ohio State University Wexner Medical Center,
6039 Varwyne Drive, Dublin, OH 43016, USA
e-mail: liz.Weinandy@osumc.edu

status, and low citrate intake. Besides increasing the amount of citrate ingested, these other factors can be altered to increase the amount of citrate excreted in the urine.

High Dietary Acid Load

Foods that increase the potential renal acid load (PRAL) of the diet increase the citrate reabsorbed by the kidney, thus decreasing the amount of citrate in the urine. Foods high in alkali, such as most fruits and vegetables, reduce the PRAL. Conversely, alkali-poor foods such as meats, poultry, eggs, and grains increase the PRAL and the risk for low urinary citrate. A diet pattern high in fruits and vegetables reduces the use of citrate as an acid buffer and allows more citrate to be excreted in the urine. As most Americans eat significant portions of grains and flesh foods, patients with low or suboptimal urine citrate should be strongly encouraged to eat moderate amounts of these foods and more ample amounts of produce. Milk, yogurt, and fats are PRAL neutral [4] (Table 6.1).

Low Carbohydrate Diets

Low carbohydrate diets are generally fruit restrictive and protein promoting which results in a higher PRAL. These diets tend to lower urinary citrate levels by causing mild metabolic acidosis and as an effect, decrease citrate excretion and increase urinary calcium excretion. These effects are greater with very low carbohydrate diets that promote ketosis. The popularity of low carbohydrate diets for weight loss raises concern for increasing the risk of kidney stones.

Low Potassium Intake

Low potassium intake and urinary potassium are associated with low urinary citrate. Hypokalemia causing intracellular acidosis increases citrate uptake and metabolism by the renal

TABLE 6.1. Average potential renal acid load (PRAL) per 100 gm edible portion.

Food group	PRAL (mEq)
Beverages	
Alkali-rich and low phosphorus	−1.7
Alkali-poor and low phosphorus	0
Fats and oils	0
Fish	7.9
Fruits and fruit juices	−3.1
Grain products	
Bread	3.5
Flour	7.0
Noodles, spaghetti	6.7
Meat and meat products	9.5
Milk and dairy products	
Milk and non-cheese products	1.0
Cheeses with lower protein content	8.0
Cheeses with higher protein content	23.6
Vegetables	−2.8

Reprinted from Remer T, Manz F. Potential renal acid load of foods and its influence on urine pH. J Am Diet Assoc. 1995;95:791–7. With permission from Elsevier

tubules, therefore impairing urinary citrate excretion [2]. Fruits and vegetables are generally good to excellent sources of potassium. Unless a patient has compromised renal function requiring potassium restriction, fruits and vegetables should be encouraged for their ability to enhance urinary citrate excretion as well as for many other health benefits.

Conditions Causing Diarrhea and Malabsorption

Chronic diarrhea and malabsorption are associated with hypocitraturia as bicarbonate wasting leads to acidosis [3]. As previously discussed, acidosis decreases urinary citrate excretion. For patients with conditions such as irritable bowel disease or short bowel syndrome, chronic diarrhea is often present, and reduced urinary citrate excretion usually results. Diarrhea is often improved through the use of a higher fiber diet and/or fiber supplements. A diet high in whole fruits and vegetables (not juices) can help manage diarrhea and also increases intake of organic acids, which are bicarbonate precursors and help normalize acid–base balance [2]. Also, some food agents like psyllium, wheat bran, and corn fiber slow the movement of food through the intestinal tract and can help control diarrhea.

Low Magnesium Status

Magnesium reduces the risk of calcium oxalate kidney stones by forming a soluble complex with oxalate. This of course will decrease the risk for crystal nucleation, aggregation, and growth of calcium oxalate stones. Furthermore, it appears that adequate oral magnesium increases the amount of urinary citrate and thus has a synergistic effect with citrate to prevent stones [5, 6]. A diet rich in high magnesium foods should be recommended, and these include green leafy vegetables, legumes, nuts, seeds, and whole grains. As many foods high in magnesium are also significant sources of oxalate, patients should be advised to consume calcium-rich foods with meals. Also, it should be noted that people with chronic diarrhea often suffer magnesium deficiencies and likely need supplemental magnesium. The Dietary Reference Intake for magnesium is 350 mg a day [7].

Citrate Intake

Citrate is not a nutrient (i.e., not essential); therefore, there is no recommended intake level. Yet, the intake of juices and foods rich in citrate appears to increase the excretion of urinary citrate. Foods generally high in citric acid are citrus fruits including lemons, limes, oranges, and grapefruits. Penniston et al. tested various fruits and found fresh lemon and lime juice to contain the greatest concentration of citrate followed by lemon and lime juice from concentrate (Fig. 6.1). Although other juices may be good sources of citrate, like orange and grapefruit juices, caution should be used when

6. Nutrition Management of Hypocitraturia

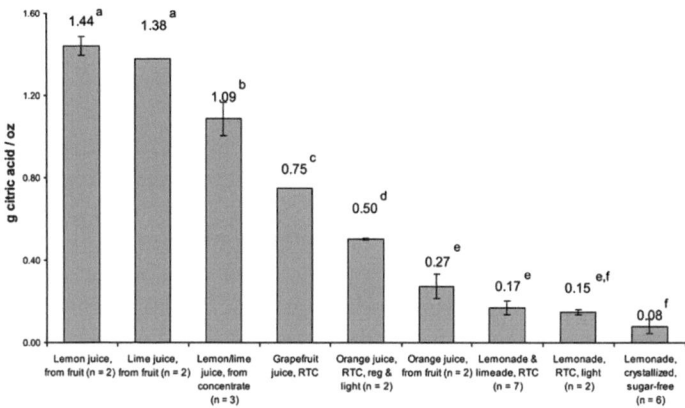

Fig. 6.1. Comparison of citric acid concentrations (g/oz.) of juices and juice products by group. [Reprinted from Penniston K, Nakada S, Holmes R, Assimos D. Quantitative assessment of citric acid in lemon juice, lime juice, and commercially-available fruit juice products. J Endourol. 2008;22(3):567–70. With permission from Mary Ann Liebert, Inc.]

recommending them as they are generally high in sugar and calories overall [8]. Studies on grapefruit juice and its effect on stone formation are mixed but large quantities should probably be limited due to its sugar and calorie content. Low sugar or "lite" variations of juices, such as lemonade, can be recommended for ease and convenience as well as improved compliance with fluid intake goals. Having patients focus on fluids with added citrate helps increase urinary citrate and total volume output (Fig. 6.1).

Summary

1. Oral citrate intake may increase urinary citrate excretion. Recommend fluids with added fresh (or from concentrate) lemon and lime juice and "lite" or "diet" lemonade. Large quantities of orange juice should be recommended with caution as it is high in sugar and calories.

2. At least five daily servings of fruits and vegetables along with smaller amounts of flesh foods and cheese discourages stone formation by lowering PRAL and increasing citrate, potassium, and magnesium intake.
3. Low urinary citrate excretion from chronic diarrhea and malabsorption can be treated with added dietary fiber and possible fiber supplements.
4. Magnesium rich foods should be consumed on a daily basis, and these include dark leafy green vegetables, legumes, nuts, seeds, and whole grains. Some of these foods may be high in oxalate. Advise patients to consume a good source of calcium with high oxalate containing foods, i.e., a container of yogurt with a spinach salad.
5. Do not advise low carbohydrate diets for weight loss. Rather, recommend a diet ample in fruits and vegetables with adequate calcium, such as the DASH diet, which also limits sodium, or other balanced weight loss diets (e.g., Weight Watchers).

References

1. Abdulhadi M, Hall P, Stree S. Hypocitraturia and its role in renal stone disease. Cleve Clin J Med. 1988;55(3):242–5.
2. Lerma E, Schwartz B. Hypocitraturia. Medscape reference [Internet]; 2013. http://emedicine.medscape.com/article/444968-overview. Cited 31 Jan 2014.
3. Zuckerman J, Assimos D. Hypocitraturia: pathophysiology and medical management. Rev Urol. 2009;11(3):134–44.
4. Remer T, Manz F. Potential renal acid load of foods and its influence on urine pH. J Am Diet Assoc. 1995;95:791–7.
5. Gershoff S, Prien E. Effect of daily MgO and vitamin B6 administration to patients with recurring calcium oxalate kidney stones. Am J Clin Nutr. 1967;20:393–9.
6. Riley J, Kim H, Averch T, Kim HJ. Effect of magnesium on calcium and oxalate ion binding. J Endourol. 2013;12:1487–92.
7. Magnesium Fact Sheet for Health Professionals [Internet]. USDA Nutrient Fact sheet, Washington (DC); 2013. http://ods.od.nih.gov/factsheets/Magnesium-HealthProfessional/. Cited 19 May 2014.
8. Penniston K, Nakada S, Holmes R, Assimos D. Quantitative assessment of citric acid in lemon juice, lime juice, and commercially-available fruit juice products. J Endourol. 2008;22(3):567–70.

Chapter 7
Medical Management of Hypocitraturia

Cynthia Denu-Ciocca

Citrate: An Inhibitor of Calcium Stone Disease

Urinary citrate is a potent endogenous inhibitor of stone formation [1, 2]. Hypocitraturia, variably defined by urinary citrate excretion <320–500 mg daily, is an important risk factor for the development of calcium kidney stones. The prevalence of hypocitraturia in different series is highly variable and ranges from approximately 20 to 60 % [3]. Citrate forms soluble complexes with calcium, decreasing the supersaturation of calcium oxalate [1]. Citrate has also been demonstrated to bind to the calcium oxalate crystal surface where it interferes with crystal growth and agglomeration [3].

Urinary Citrate Excretion

Urinary citrate excretion is determined by multiple factors. The acid–base status of a particular individual has the strongest influence on urinary citrate excretion. Metabolic acidosis and dietary acid loads increase proximal tubular reabsorption

C. Denu-Ciocca, MD (✉)
Kidney Center, University of North Carolina at Chapel Hill,
7006 Burnett Womack, CB 7155, Chapel Hill, NC 27599, USA
e-mail: cynthia_denu-ciocca@med.unc.edu

M. Monga et al. (eds.), *Pocket Guide to Kidney Stone Prevention*, DOI 10.1007/978-3-319-11098-1_7, of citrate, a potential base, leading to decreased urinary citrate excretion. Alkalemia induces the opposite effect, promoting increased citrate excretion. Most often hypocitraturia is idiopathic; however, certain medical conditions are associated with decreased citrate excretion. These disorders include distal renal tubular acidosis, hypokalemia, and gastrointestinal malabsorption due to bowel resection, bariatric surgery, and pancreatic insufficiency. Medications, including carbonic anhydrase inhibitors such as topiramate, are also associated with reduced citrate excretion.

Citrate Therapy

Treatment with citrate preparations is one of the few evidence-based interventions proven to reduce recurring stones in patients with recurrent stone disease, particularly in stone formers with hypocitraturia [4, 5]. Citrate provides an alkali load which subsequently leads to increased urinary citrate excretion. Citrate therapy also increases urinary pH which is an important component of the treatment of uric acid and cystine stones. Prospective randomized controlled trials have evaluated the efficacy of various alkali citrate preparations for the prevention of recurrent calcium nephrolithiasis [6–8]. Treatment with potassium citrate and potassium–magnesium citrate therapy resulted in significant reductions in recurrent stone disease [7, 8]. However, Hofbauer and colleagues failed to show any significant reduction in recurrence in calcium stone formers treated with sodium-potassium citrate compared to matched controls [6]. This may be related to the effect of sodium to increase urinary calcium excretion. Potassium citrate has also been effective in patients who did not have hypocitraturia; it may therefore be appropriate when urine chemistries are relatively unremarkable or when other therapeutic options have not been effective.

Two prospective, randomized studies have shown significantly lower rates of stone recurrence and growth of residual stone fragments in patients treated with alkali citrate prophylaxis for 1 year after shock wave lithotripsy and/or percutaneous nephrolithotomy [9, 10]. A dramatic reduction in stone recurrence was demonstrated in one controlled study when subjects who were stone-free after lithotripsy received medical prophylaxis [9]. None of the subjects treated with potassium citrate 60 meq/day had recurrent stones after 12 months compared to 28.5 % in those who did not receive prophylactic treatment. Medically treated patients with residual stone fragments also had lower rates of stone growth compared to the untreated group [9]. Lojanapiwat et al. [10] studied the effect of sodium-potassium citrate on stone recurrence and regrowth after either shockwave lithotripsy or percutaneous nephrolithotomy in patients who were stone-free or had residual stone burden. After 12 months both stone-free status and unchanged stone size were significantly more frequent in the medical prophylaxis group compared to matched controls. For patients who were rendered stone-free, there was a 5.3-fold relative risk for recurrence in the control group compared to the medical prophylaxis group. Patients who had residual stone fragments were 1.38-fold more likely to have growth of their residual stones.

Although different forms of citrate have been shown to benefit calcium stone formers, potassium citrate is the preferred therapy. The potassium content of this preparation provides the advantage of potentially preventing hypokalemia often associated with concomitant thiazide use. This benefit is significant because hypokalemia mediates hypocitraturia and may limit thiazide efficacy. Furthermore, sodium–potassium citrate may diminish the benefit of citrate therapy as urinary sodium promotes increased calcium excretion.

Potassium citrate is available in tablet, crystals (for dissolution), and liquid forms. Tablets are available in a long-release wax matrix form in doses of 5, 10, and 15 meq. The wax matrix may appear in the toilet after bowel movements without implying that the medication was not effective or not absorbed; patients should be warned about this possibility to prevent unnecessary telephone calls to the office. However, the tablet forms may not be absorbed as well as the liquid preparations in patients with malabsorptive states and higher transit times. Crystals, when available, come in 30 meq packets and can be given as ½–1 packet twice a day. Liquid preparations are usually 1 meq/mL, so that typical doses would be 1–2 tablespoons (15–30 ml) twice a day. Potassium citrate therapy is generally well tolerated, but is associated with gastrointestinal side effects that include dyspepsia, nausea, vomiting, diarrhea, GI mucosal injury, and GI obstruction. Potassium citrate is therefore contraindicated in patients with delayed gastric emptying, intestinal obstruction, and peptic ulcer disease. A 25 meq effervescent tablet of potassium bicarbonate, dissolved in water, may be better tolerated for some patients; the alkali load is associated with an increase in citrate excretion. Patients with advanced chronic kidney disease, as well as individuals on potassium-sparing diuretics or medications that inhibit the renin–angiotensin–aldosterone system are at increased risk for hyperkalemia. Sodium citrate or sodium bicarbonate may be prescribed as alternative therapies to the potassium-based alkali in patients at risk for hyperkalemia, those who are unable to tolerate potassium citrate or for stone formers in which cost is prohibitive. Sodium citrate comes in a solution that contains 1 meq/mL or 1 meq of bicarbonate equivalent, with citric acid added for palatability. Citric acid, like any organic acid, is neutral with respect to acid–base balance, as it yields a bicarbonate ion during hepatic metabolism, effectively neutralizing its attendant proton. Sodium bicarbonate can be given as baking soda, with ¼ teaspoon containing about 14 meq of sodium and bicarbonate each, and in 650 mg or roughly 8 meq tabs. Disadvantages of sodium containing citrate preparations include increased urinary calcium excretion. Worsening hypervolemia in patients with congestive heart failure and advanced chronic kidney disease, as well as exacerbation of hypertension in individuals who are salt-sensitive, are very infrequent.

Dosing of alkali depends on the severity of the metabolic acidosis and hypocitraturia. Typically citrate may be initiated at doses of 40–60 meq/day in divided doses. Patients who suffer from distal renal tubular acidosis often need higher doses of potassium citrate due to extreme hypocitraturia and hypokalemia. Dosing should be adjusted based on results of serum electrolytes, urine pH, and the 24-h urine metabolic indices.

Monitoring of serum potassium is generally recommended approximately 7–30 days after initiating or modifying the dose of potassium citrate, particularly in those with CKD or who are taking angiotensin converting enzyme inhibitors and angiotensin receptor blockers.

Another potential concern in alkali treatment is that the resultant higher urinary pH may promote calcium phosphate stone formation, or convert calcium oxalate stone formers to calcium phosphate stone formers. Calcium phosphate stones have become more prevalent and pose a treatment dilemma because up to one third of these patients present with large stones and bilateral disease. The importance of this possible effect remains uncertain. Although alkali citrate therapy has been suggested to increase the propensity to form calcium phosphate stones, it may also prevent these stones. However, there are no prospective randomized controlled trails to assess the effect of citrate therapy in calcium phosphate stone formers. Patients who suffer from distal renal tubular acidosis are unable to acidify their urine and subsequently have high baseline urine pH. These patients typically produce predominantly calcium phosphate stones. A non-randomized study in subjects with recurrent calcium nephrolithiasis due to distal renal tubular acidosis demonstrated a significant decrease in stone recurrence after treatment with potassium citrate despite their preexisting alkaline urine pH [4]. Further studies are required to prospectively evaluate the potential benefit of citrate therapy in reducing stone calcium phosphate stone recurrence. The likelihood of increasing the risk of calcium phosphate stones is minimized if fluid intake is kept high and, in some cases, if thiazides limit hypercalciuria.

Summary

- Citrate is a potent inhibitor of stone formation and urinary citrate excretion of less than 320–500 mg daily is termed hypocitraturia.
- Hypocitraturia is an important risk factor for the development of kidney stones with a prevalence of 20–60 %.

- Citrate decreases free urinary calcium and inhibits crystal nucleation, growth, and aggregation.
- Urinary citrate excretion is determined by multiple factors but acid–base status has the largest impact.
- Most patients have idiopathic hypocitraturia however medical disease including distal renal tubular acidosis, hypokalemia, and gastrointestinal malabsorption are common causes for reduced citrate excretion.
- Medications including carbonic anhydrase inhibitors such as topiramate are also associated with reduced citrate excretion.
- Therapy with citrate has been demonstrated to reduce the risk of recurrent calcium stones in hypocitraturic stone formers and those with normal citrate excretion. Potassium citrate is the preferred form of citrate therapy and potentially may prevent hypokalemia associated with concomitant thiazide administration.
- Sodium citrate and sodium bicarbonate may be utilized to increase citrate excretion in patients unable to tolerate or afford potassium citrate.

References

1. Kok DJ, Papapoulos SE, Bijvoet OL. Excessive crystal agglomeration with low citrate excretion in recurrent stone-formers. Lancet. 1986;10(1):1056–8.
2. Ryall RL. Urinary inhibitors of calcium oxalate crystallization and their potential role in stone formation. World J Urol. 1997;15(3):155–64.
3. Zuckerman JM, Assimos DG. Hypocitraturia: pathophysiology and medical management. Rev Urol. 2009;11(3):134–44.
4. Preminger GM, Sakhaee K, Skurla C, Pak CY. Prevention of recurrent calcium stone formation with potassium citrate therapy in patients with distal renal tubular acidosis. J Urol. 1985;134(1):20–3.
5. Pak CY, Fuller C. Idiopathic hypocitraturic calcium-oxalate nephrolithiasis successfully treated with potassium citrate. Ann Intern Med. 1986;104(1):33–7.

6. Hofbauer J, Höbarth K, Szabo N, Marberger M. Alkali citrate prophylaxis in idiopathic recurrent calcium oxalate urolithiasis—a prospective randomized study. Br J Urol. 1994;73(4):362–5.
7. Ettinger B, Pak CY, Citron JT, Thomas C, Adams-Huet B, Vangessel A. Potassium–magnesium citrate is an effective prophylaxis against recurrent calcium oxalate nephrolithiasis. J Urol. 1997;158(6):2069–73.
8. Barcelo P, Wuhl O, Servitge E, Rousaud A, Pak CY. Randomized double-blind study of potassium citrate in idiopathic hypocitraturic calcium nephrolithiasis. J Urol. 1993;150(6):1761–4.
9. Soygür T, Akbay A, Küpeli S. Effect of potassium citrate therapy on stone recurrence and residual fragments after shockwave lithotripsy in lower caliceal calcium oxalate urolithiasis: a randomized controlled trial. J Endourol. 2002;16(3):149–52.
10. Lojanapiwat B, Tanthanuch M, Pripathanont C, Ratchanon S, Srinualnad S, Taweemonkongsap T, et al. Alkaline citrate reduces stone recurrence and regrowth after shockwave lithotripsy and percutaneous nephrolithotomy. Int Braz J Urol. 2011;37(5):611–6.

Chapter 8
Nutritional Management of Hyperoxaluria

Kristina L. Penniston

Introduction

Oxalate is both consumed and produced by humans. It is consumed as either the organic acid (oxalic acid) or as a "salt" (e.g., potassium oxalate, sodium oxalate, calcium oxalate). Oxalate is not a nutrient; it is not required for life. While plants, fungi, and algae produce and have use for it, there is no known use for oxalate by humans. In fact, oxalate has historically been known as an "anti-nutrient" due to its ability to bind with calcium, magnesium, zinc, iron, and other essential minerals in the gastrointestinal (GI) tract and reduce their absorption, contributing to mineral deficiency. After it is produced in vivo or absorbed from the GI tract, oxalate must be excreted. Dermal excretion of oxalate is not described. Excretion is therefore handled by the renal system. When urine oxalate is high, or when its excretion is not adequately opposed by crystal inhibitors, it complexes with available urinary calcium and magnesium. While magnesium oxalate is quite soluble in urine,

K.L. Penniston, PhD, RD (✉)
Department of Urology, University of Wisconsin, School of Medicine and Public Health, 1685 Highland Ave., 3258 Medical Foundation Centennial Building, Madison, WI 53705-2281, USA
e-mail: penn@urology.wisc.edu

calcium oxalate is not. High urine oxalate is thus a risk factor for calcium oxalate stone formation.

Urinary oxalate excretion is normally between five and tenfold lower than calcium (mg/mg). The rate of change of calcium oxalate supersaturation is calculated to be 10–23 times greater for oxalate than calcium [1]. Accordingly, many argue that urine oxalate should be considered a continuous vs. a dichotomous variable. Indeed, a small increase in urinary oxalate excretion can significantly increase calcium oxalate stone risk. However, as not all patients who form calcium oxalate stones demonstrate high urine oxalate, other factors are important, such as urine volume, urinary citrate excretion, and urinary calcium excretion. These factors are addressed in other chapters.

General Nutritional Management of High Urine Oxalate

Nutritional management of high urine oxalate requires the identification of modifiable risk factors and begins with a full assessment of habitual dietary intake, overall dietary pattern, supplement use, and medical history. There are currently few pharmacologic approaches to managing hyperoxaluria. Dietary measures are employed to address the biosynthesis, absorption, and urinary concentration and solubility of oxalate, depending on which of these is thought to be contributory to high urine oxalate (Fig. 8.1).

As with other medical conditions, treatment of the underlying cause(s) or contributor(s) is recommended. With dietary recommendations, the tendency is often to provide *all* recommendations to *all* patients, regardless of variable dietary contributions and, often, without regard to how the patient may already be eating. Few other medical therapies encourage such a "blanket" approach to medical management. Nutrition therapy for stones is best applied when targeted to address a specific dietary cause(s) for a patient's increased

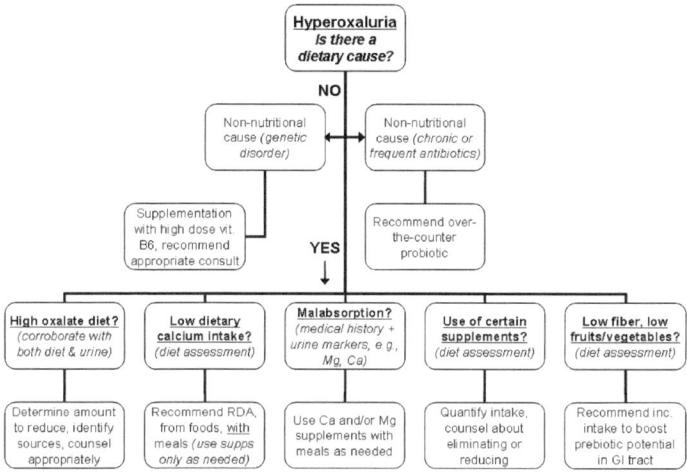

Fig. 8.1. Decision tool and guide for the dietary management of high urine oxalate. [Reprinted from Penniston KL, Nakada SY. Diet and alternative therapies in the management of stone disease. Urol Clin North Am. 2013;40(1):31–46. With permission from Elsevier]

stone risk. Some means of assessing patients' current diets are usually required in order to determine whether there are contributors to stone risk factors. If dietary factors are well-controlled despite the persistence of biochemical aberration(s), then non-dietary etiologies are considered.

Controlling Oxalate Biosynthesis

There is no medication to reduce oxalate synthesis. For patients with one of the three known variants of primary hyperoxaluria (PH), a combined liver/kidney transplant corrects overproduction of oxalate by eliminating the respective enzyme deficiency or dysfunction. The subset of patients with PH type 1 who are deficient in alanine-glyoxylate aminotransferase (AGXT) may respond favorably to supraphysiologic doses of vitamin B6 (pyridoxine), 100–500 mg/day [2].

The vitamin is a co-enzyme for AGXT, which converts glyoxylic acid to glycine, thus diverting it away from oxalate production. But patients with a functional absence of AGXT would not be expected to benefit from vitamin B6 supplementation as even the highest of co-enzyme concentrations would be useless in the setting of complete enzyme inactivity.

Recently, reduced urinary oxalate excretion in patients with idiopathic hyperoxaluria has been reported with vitamin B6 [3]. Deficiency is very uncommon in the US and in other developed nations, and it is therefore unlikely that vitamin B6 deficiency accounts in any appreciable way for hyperoxaluria. However, with 146 known AGXT mutations [4] and possibly more yet undiscovered, patients with subtle forms of undiagnosed PH could exist due to mutations that may interfere with cofactor binding [5]. In this scenario, vitamin B6 supplementation could be useful in ramping up enzyme activity rendered abnormal due to a mutation. This may explain the favorable effects from pyridoxine observed in some, but not all, patients with idiopathic hyperoxaluria.

Controlling GI Oxalate Absorption

Oxalate is absorbed throughout the GI tract, mostly in the small intestine. Typically, only 5–10 % of the oxalate consumed is absorbed. This is due, in part, to the fact that much of the oxalate consumed is in the form of insoluble oxalate, e.g., calcium oxalate. Evidence in the literature supports the appropriate use of dietary calcium and, to a lesser extent, magnesium, as a way to control oxalate absorption [6]. When oxalate binds with these and other divalent cations in the GI tract, an insoluble complex is formed, resulting in the absorption of neither constituent. The amount of calcium or other mineral required to bind a known amount of oxalate varies depending on the form in which the oxalate was initially consumed, on the presence and type of dietary fats, on GI transit time, and other factors.

Role of Calcium and Magnesium

Assuming normal GI functioning, the Recommended Dietary Allowance (RDA) for calcium, in the range of 1,000–1,300 mg/day (depending on gender and life-stage group), is sufficient to provide optimal GI binding potential for oxalate. Most evidence recommends this be distributed more-or-less equally at meals throughout the day; but other data suggest that intake need not be divided at meals [7]. Calcium from foods and beverages, as opposed to supplements, is strongly recommended as it is difficult to consume excessive calcium from diet alone. A multitude of dietary calcium sources exist, both dairy and non-dairy (Table 8.1). The RDA for adults for

TABLE 8.1. Calcium content of some foods and beverages providing >100 mg calcium per typical household serving (footnotes categorize as dairy or non-dairy, lactose-free or lactose-containing).

Food item	Amount	Calcium (mg)
Calcium-fortified, ready-to-consume breakfast cereals[a]	1 cup (30–50 g, depending on cereal)	Can be up to 1,000
Tofu, firm, processed with calcium[a]	½ cup (about 124 g)	430
Calcium-fortified orange and other fruit juices[a]	1 cup (8 fluid ozs; 240 mL)	300–500
Calcium-fortified non-dairy milks (rice, soy, almond, coconut, flaxseed, hemp)[a]	1 cup (8 fluid ozs; 240 mL)	300–450 (brands vary)
Dairy milk (cow, goat, camel)[a]	1 cup (8 fluid ozs; 240 mL)	300–400
Kefir (made from cow, goat, or sheep milk)[b]	1 cup (8 fluid ozs; 240 mL)	300
Buttermilk[b]	1 cup (8 fluid ozs; 240 mL)	285
Cheese[b]	1 oz (about 28 g)	200–400 (varies by type)
Yogurt (made from cow, goat, or sheep milk)[b]	6–8 ozs	180–450 (varies by brand and formulation)
Blackstrap molasses[a]	1 tablespoon (about 15 mL)	170

(continued)

TABLE 8.1. (continued)

Food item	Amount	Calcium (mg)
Non-dairy calcium-fortified yogurt (e.g., rice, soy almond, coconut)[a]	6–8 ozs	150–500 (varies by brand and formulation)
Canned sardines, in oil, with bones[a]	1 oz (about 28 g)	105
Kale, dandelion greens, turnip greens, okra[a]	1 cup, chopped (about 34 g)	100–140
Whey protein powder[c]	1 oz (about 28 g)	100–120 (formulations vary)
Figs, dried[a]	8 whole	100

[a]Non-dairy, lactose-free
[b]Dairy, but lactose is reduced due to microbial fermentation
[c]Derived from dairy, but most of the lactose is removed during separation from milk

magnesium is in the range of 310–420 mg/day; multiple dietary sources are available to meet this need. In patients with already appropriate calcium and magnesium intakes, further investigation to determine the contributor(s) to high urine oxalate is required.

Controlling GI Oxalate Concentration

The concentration of oxalate along the GI tract may be directly related to the amount of oxalate absorbed. Strategies to reduce the GI concentration of oxalate include optimizing bacterial oxalate degradation, controlling oxalate intake, and controlling fat malabsorption.

Bacterial Oxalate Degradation

Oxalate is substrate for multiple bacteria, including those which use other substrate, and results in the production of carbon dioxide and formate. Oxalobacter *formigenes* is a common inhabitant of the mammalian GI tract and is an obligate oxalate user. More than a dozen other bacteria are known to degrade oxalate in humans, including some enterococcus, lactobacillus, streptococcus, and bifidobacterium species. Given that humans have long depended on bacteria to regulate oxalate degradation, it makes sense that a healthy gut "microbiome" (outnumbering the host's own genes 150-fold) [8] could reduce oxalate absorption and urinary excretion. However, disruptions in the host-microbe environment are common and may include antibiotic use, a diet suboptimal for prebiotic material (foods providing non-digestible matter required by bacteria as substrate), altered GI physiology, and inflammatory bowel diseases, especially those that shorten gut transit time.

If dysbiosis is suspected as a contributor to high urine oxalate, a diet rich in prebiotics (as from fruits, vegetables, and high fiber grains) to maintain healthy gut flora, regular ingestion of foods with live bacterial cultures, and, in some cases, probiotic supplements, may be recommended. As data are variable with respect to the specific bacterial species and probiotic formulations most effective in reducing urine oxalate [9], there are no agreed-upon clinical recommendations.

Oxalate Intake

Dietary oxalate restriction is controversial. No controlled trials have demonstrated reduced calcium oxalate stone formation with a low-oxalate diet. Limiting or reducing oxalate intake should be reserved only for patients whose intake of oxalate is assessed as high AND is unopposed by an appropriate intake of calcium. Foods highest in oxalate are often those richest for fiber, magnesium, phytate, and antioxidants—all of which may inhibit calcium stone formation by various mechanisms. Moreover, the concentration of oxalate in a food does not always correlate with its bioavailability, which is dependent on the form of oxalate in the food as well as on the other nutritional components consumed at the same time from other foods, as in a meal. Consider dietary recommendations to control blood glucose in people with diabetes. The carbohydrate content of a single food item is not so much stressed as is balancing carbohydrate intake with protein, fiber, and fat. In similar fashion, perhaps patients should be encouraged to consume oxalate-containing foods — most of which are healthy and nutritious — within a balanced meal setting, especially one providing calcium.

Fat Malabsorption

Urinary oxalate excretion may be high due to fat malabsorption, the presence of undigested and unabsorbed fat in the large intestine. Normally, fat is digested and fatty acids are absorbed prior to reaching the large intestine. In intestinal malabsorption, unabsorbed fatty acids complex with calcium and magnesium. This increases the concentration of free oxalate in the digestive tract because less calcium and magnesium are available to bind it. Thus, in patients with fat malabsorption, frequent calcium and/or magnesium supplementation with meals may be required to ensure adequate oxalate binding. Alternatively, or in addition, nutritional interventions to address the primary cause of the malabsorption are employed.

Finally, a role for fish oil providing docosahexanoic and eicosapentoic fatty acids (DHA and EPA, respectively) has been postulated. While further research is warranted, not only to prove clinical efficacy but to identify mechanism(s) of action, dosages of 1,500 mg of DHA+EPA daily may be tried [10].

Summary

- Determine if diet is contributory to high urine oxalate; if so, identify why (Fig. 8.1).
- If low calcium intake is assessed in the setting of hyperoxaluria, recommend calcium-containing foods and/or beverages at each meal, providing 300–400 mg, to enhance oxalate binding in the GI tract.

- If high-oxalate intake is assessed, recommend calcium-containing foods and/or beverages at each meal to enhance oxalate binding potential in the GI tract and/or recommend reduced intake of specific high-oxalate foods.
- If suboptimal bacterial oxalate degradation is assessed, recommend (a) increased intake of foods/beverages providing live bacterial cultures to enhance bacterial oxalate degradation, and/or (b) probiotic supplementation.
- If fruit/vegetable intake is <5 servings/day, recommend increasing to provide prebiotic material to support and sustain healthy gut flora capable of degrading oxalate.
- If vitamin B6 insufficiency/deficiency or suboptimal enzyme activity is suspected, recommend pyridoxine supplementation, typically in the range of 100–200 mg/day.
- If fat malabsorption is assessed as the driving factor for high urine oxalate, dietary measures to address malabsorption should be recommended and may include: higher fiber intake, replacement of divalent cations that are made unavailable for oxalate binding due to the formation of fatty acid soaps, correction of dysbiosis (if present), and other strategies (e.g., pancreatic enzymes in the setting of pancreatic insufficiency, reduced fat intake in the setting of gallbladder insufficiency).
- Fish oil, providing 1,500 mg daily of EPA+DHA, may be recommended.

References

1. Rodgers A. Aspects of calcium oxalate crystallization: theory, in vitro studies, and in vivo implementation. J Am Soc Nephrol. 1999;14:S351–4.
2. Mitwalli A, Ayiomamitis A, Grass L, Oreopoulos DG. Control of hyperoxaluria with large doses of pyridoxine in patients with kidney stones. Int Urol Nephrol. 1988;20:353–9.
3. Ortiz-Alvarado O, Miyaoka R, Kriedberg C, Moeding A, Stessman M, Monga M. Pyridoxine and dietary counseling for the management of idiopathic hyperoxaluria in stone-forming patients. Urology. 2011;77:1054–8.

4. Williams EL, Acquaviva C, Amoroso A, Chevalier F, Coulter-Mackie M, Monico CG, Giachino D, Owen T, Robbiano A, Salido E, Waterham H, Rumsby G. Primary hyperoxaluria type 1: update and additional mutation analysis of the AGXT gene. Hum Mutat. 2009;30:910–7.
5. Ames BN, Elson-Schwab I, Silver EA. High-dose vitamin therapy stimulates variant enzymes with decreased coenzyme binding affinity (increased K_m): relevance to genetic disease and polymorphisms. Am J Clin Nutr. 2002;75:616–58.
6. Penniston KL, Nakada SY. Diet and alternative therapies in the management of stone disease. Urol Clin North Am. 2013;40:31–46.
7. Lange JN, Wood KD, Mufarrij PW, Callahan MF, Easter L, Knight J, Holmes RP, Assimos DG. The impact of dietary calcium and oxalate ratios on stone risk. J Urol. 2012;79:1226–9.
8. Wu GD, Lewis JD. Analysis of the human gut microbiome and association with disease. Clin Gastroenterol Hepatol. 2013;7:774–7.
9. Liebman M, Al-Wahsh IA. Probiotics and other key determinants of dietary oxalate absorption. Adv Nutr. 2011;2:254–60.
10. Siener R, Jansen B, Watzer B, Hesse A. Effect of n-3 fatty acid supplementation on urinary risk factors for calcium oxalate stone formation. J Urol. 2011;185:719–24.

Part III
Uric Acid Stones

Chapter 9
Nutrition Management of Uric Acid Stones

Lisa A. Davis

Nutrition management of uric acid stone disease begins with a full assessment of dietary and fluid intakes (including beverages containing alcohol and fructose), dietary patterns, supplement use, weight, and medical history to identify modifiable risk factors.

Fluids

Increased fluid intake is a common recommendation for all stone formers. Low urine volume can be the result of insufficient intake, gastrointestinal and insensible losses. While there is no agreement on the total amount of fluid that should be consumed, it is recommended to consume enough fluid to produce at least 2 L of urine daily to maintain suitably low urine uric acid supersaturation.

L.A. Davis, MS, RD (✉)
Clinical Research Unit, University of Wisconsin Institute
for Clinical and Translational Research,
Clinical Science Center, F4/120, 600 Highland Avenue,
Madison, WI 53792, USA
e-mail: ldavis5@uwhealth.org

Protein

Uric acid is derived from two primary sources, endogenous production in the liver and dietary ingestion of purines. The dietary input to uric acid biosynthesis varies among uric acid stone formers. Because human tissues lack the enzyme uricase to metabolize purines, the end product, uric acid, must be eliminated by the gut and the kidneys. As a result of this relationship, nutrition therapy has focused on limiting foods containing purines, namely, protein from animal sources [1]. While flesh proteins such as red meats, poultry, and fish contain high amounts of purines, dairy products contain minimal purines. In uric acid stone formers with a high intake of non-dairy animal foods, nutrition therapy should be aimed at avoiding excessive intake of such foods on a daily basis. In addition, foods particularly high in purine content such as organ meats, sweetbreads (thymus and pancreas glands), fish and shellfish, beef, pork, poultry, and fowl should be limited [2].

Plant-based foods are also known to contain purines. While asparagus, cauliflower, beans, lentils, mushrooms, oatmeal, peas, and spinach are sometimes limited due to their relatively high purine content, the amount and type of purines vary as well as their bioavailability for conversion to uric acid. Plant-based purines and low fat dairy products have not been associated with increased uric acid concentration nor the risk of gout in men [3, 4]. As gout is a condition of excessive uric acid biosynthesis, these data have been used to support no limit on plant-based purine sources in uric acid stone formers.

Alcohol

Alcohol consumption is known to increase the serum concentration of uric acid. In addition alcoholic beverages contain purines, and beer contains a higher proportion of purines relative to other alcoholic beverages [5]. Alcohol intake has been directly related to uric acid level and the risk of gout in men; however, gout risk varied according to the type of alcoholic beverage consumed. While beer and liquor intake were both associated with risk of gout, beer consumption was linked to a higher risk of gout than liquor; wine consumption was not associated with gout risk [6]. No studies have determined the association between alcohol consumption and uric acid stone risk. Although it has not been determined whether alcohol should be restricted or one type of beverage should be recommended over another, it seems reasonable to adhere to general healthy diet recommendations to limit all types of alcoholic beverages to one per day.

Urine Acidity

Dietary intake has the potential to alter the pH of the urinary environment. Sulfate, a major determinant of daily acid load, is derived from the oxidation of sulfur-containing amino acids found in animal proteins and cereal grains. Persons consuming diets rich in animal and cereal protein excrete higher amounts of sulfate, phosphate, and uric acid compared to persons eating plant-based/vegetarian diets rich in fruits and vegetables, resulting in greater net acid excretion and more acidic urinary pH. Potassium, found in fruits and vegetables, contributes dietary base which can neutralize acid load of the diet [7].

While a 24-h urine analysis is necessary to directly measure net acid excretion, two methods are available for estimating the effect of diet-related endogenous acid production; both methods require a food record or a diet recall and analysis of micronutrient intake. Net acid excretion can be determined indirectly by subtracting the sum of urinary cations (sodium, potassium, calcium, and magnesium) from the sum of urinary anions (chloride, phosphorus, sulfate, and organic acids). Values for the potential renal acid load (PRAL) of single foods have been published, and average values have been calculated for food groups as well. Positive PRAL values indicate the availability of excess acid forming potential; cheese, meat, poultry, fish, eggs, and grains generate positive values. Negative PRAL values, generated by fruits and vegetables, moderate the potential for acid production. Fat, milk, and non-cheese products exert a neutral effect on acid production [8]. Diets high in energy, animal protein, and alcohol produce higher, positive PRAL values as compared to lacto-ovo vegetarian diets. Diets lower in protein and using a combination of animal and vegetable proteins fall midway between the two in terms of urinary pH and PRAL [7]. The merit of PRAL lies in its usefulness for assessing the acid forming potential of individual meals and habitual dietary patterns and their contribution to urine acidity.

Similar to PRAL the ratio of protein and potassium can be used to estimate the balance between protein-containing foods and fruits and vegetables and to predict acid load of the diet [9].

Fructose

Fructose intake from added sugars, fruits, and fruit juices has been associated with increased kidney stone risk [10]. Rising rates of obesity, metabolic syndrome, and diabetes parallel the increase in fructose consumption. Although studies have not specifically linked fructose to uric acid stones, fructose is thought to exert its effect through increased uric acid production. Insulin resistance may also play a contributing role [11]. While data are limited, nutrition recommendations should target excessive intakes of foods and beverages sweetened with high fructose corn syrup. This may help to maintain a healthy body weight as obesity is associated with acidic urine.

Obesity, Diabetes, and Metabolic Syndrome

Obesity, type 2 diabetes mellitus, and metabolic syndrome are emerging as risk factors for uric acid stone formation. In addition, low urine pH has been noted among uric acid stone formers who are obese and who exhibit features of the metabolic syndrome. Although the mechanism is unclear, current research suggests insulin resistance may play a role in altered renal ammoniagenesis and/or excretion resulting in impaired acid buffering which contributes to persistently acidic urine [12]. Interventions targeting insulin resistance, such as weight control, exercise, and the use of insulin or oral glycemic control agents, have not been studied with respect to the prevention/recurrence of uric acid stones. However, it seems reasonable to incorporate good blood sugar control in addition to other measures as needed to reduce the risk of uric acid stone formation.

Other Dietary Modifications

Uric acid may serve as the nidus for calcium oxalate stones. Please see the chapter on calcium oxalate for additional dietary recommendations to prevent stone formation.

Summary

No research to date suggests that nutrition modifications will prevent the formation of new stones; however, lifestyle modifications have the potential to affect serum uric acid levels and alter the urinary environment. To summarize, if urinary uric acid excretion is high and/or if urine pH is low, recommend:

- Enough fluid to produce a minimum of 2 L of urine daily
- Limit foods containing high amounts of purines
- Limit the total amount of flesh proteins
- Encourage a diet rich in fruits and vegetables
- Limit alcohol to a maximum of one drink daily
- Encourage healthy body weight or weight loss to achieve healthy body weight.

References

1. Best SL. Protein restriction and stone disease: myth or reality? In: Pearle MS, Nakada SY, editors. Practical controversies in medical management of stone disease. New York: Springer Science+Business Media; 2014. p. 71–90.
2. Tracy CF, Best S, Bagrodia A, Poindexter JR, Adams-Huet B, Sakhaee K, Maalouf N, Pak CYC, Pearle MS. Animal protein and the risk of kidney stones: a comparative metabolic study of animal protein sources. J Urol. 2014;192:137–41.
3. Choi HK, Atkinson K, Karlson EW, Willett W, Curhan G. Purine-rich foods, dairy and protein intake, and the risk of gout in men. N Engl J Med. 2004;350:1093–103.
4. Zgaga L, Theodoratou E, Kyle J, Farrington SM, Agakov F, Tenesa A, Walker M, McNeill G, Wright AF, Rudan I, Dunlop MG, Campbell H. The association of dietary intake of purine-rich vegetables, sugar-sweetened beverages and dairy with plasma urate, in a cross-sectional study. PLoS One. 2012;7(6):e38123.
5. Yamamoto T, Moriwaki Y, Takahashi S. Effect of ethanol on metabolism of purine bases (hypoxanthine, xanthine, and uric acid). Clin Chim Acta. 2005;356:35–57.
6. Choi HK, Curhan G. Beer, liquor, and wine consumption and uric acid level: the third national health and nutrition examination survey. Arthritis Rheum. 2004;51:1023–9.
7. Adeva MM, Souto G. Diet-induced metabolic acidosis. Clin Nutr. 2011;30:416–21.
8. Remer T, Manz F. Potential renal acid load of foods and its influence on urine pH. J Am Diet Assoc. 1995;95:791–7.
9. Frassetto LA, Todd KM, Morris Jr RC, Sebastian A. Estimation of net endogenous noncarbonic acid production in humans from diet potassium and protein contents. Am J Clin Nutr. 1998;68:576–83.
10. Taylor EN, Curhan GC. Fructose consumption and the risk of kidney stones. Kidney Int. 2008;73:207–2012.
11. Johnson RJ, Nakagawa T, Sanchez-Lozada LG, Shafiu M, Sundaram S, Le M, Ishimoto T, Sautin YY, Lanaspa MA. Sugar, uric acid, and the etiology of diabetes and obesity. Diabetes. 2013;62:3307–15.
12. Maalouf NM. Metabolic syndrome and the genesis of uric acid stones. J Ren Nutr. 2011;21:128–31.

Chapter 10
Medical Management of Uric Acid Stones

John S. Rodman

General Principles

- Uric acid is a weak organic acid whose solubility at pH 6.5 is approximately 11 times greater than at pH 5.0. Hence, uric acid stones will usually form only when the urinary pH is low most or all of the time.
- Normally the pH of the urine rises after a meal. Parietal cells in the stomach form hydrochloric acid and transiently leave base in the blood which spills into the urine and dissolves any uric acid crystals which may have formed [1].
- Uric acid stone formers lose this post-prandial alkaline tide which protects against uric acid crystal formation. Alkaline salt therapy will often dissolve a pure uric acid calculus as long as there is free flow of urine past the stone.

J.S. Rodman, MD (✉)
Department of Medicine/Nephrology, Weill Cornell School of Medicine, 435 East 57 Street, New York, NY 10022, USA
e-mail: jrodmanmd@aol.com

Situations Which Lead to a Persistently Acid Urine

1. A defect in ammonia production requiring the kidney to use the phosphate buffer pair to excrete most of the acid load by keeping the urine pH low. This defect is frequently age related and is one reason uric acid stones are more common in patients over the age of 50.
2. Obesity, diabetes, and the metabolic syndrome. Patients with insulin resistance have a defect in ammoniagenesis [2].
3. A diet high in animal protein, the chief source of non-volatile acid the kidney must excrete.
4. A ketogenic diet which is deliberately restricted in carbohydrate content.
5. Lower gastrointestinal losses of base. Chronic diarrhea, whether from bowel disease, drugs such as mestinon (myasthenia gravis), or sertraline (depression).

Types of Bowel Disease

The prototype of intestinal dysfunction causing uric acid stones is the patient with an ileostomy. Lack of colonic function results in loss of base and results in an increased acid load that the kidney must excrete. Any situation which leads to an increase in stool volume can have the same effect. On the other hand, the patient with a small bowel resection for Crohn's disease usually makes calcium oxalate stones. Malabsorption of fat leads to precipitation of divalent cations in the proximal bowel allowing oxalate to escape to the distal part of the GI tract where this anion is hyper-absorbed. To be sure, both types of GI problems can co-exist but the distinction is frequently useful.

10. Medical Management of Uric Acid Stones   83

Other Factors

1. Dehydration is a risk factor for all types of stones. Some patients make pure uric acid stones only when traveling to hot climates. Hikers or skiers at high altitudes such as the Rocky Mountains will lose large amounts of water without realizing it because perspiration does not accumulate. Travelers may avoid fluids because of the nuisance of finding a bathroom.
2. A high protein diet not only increases the amount of nonvolatile acid the kidney must excrete. It also increases the purine load. Glandular meats, sausages and gravies are the worst.
3. Rapid weight loss increases the uric acid to be excreted.
4. Catabolic states and chemotherapy may also increase uric acid excretion. Occasionally, a first uric acid stone can be the harbinger of a small cell tumor of the lung or other malignancy.
5. Uricosuric drugs can lead to uric acid stone formation particularly when they are initiated for gout treatment. Probenecid increases uric acid excretion but reduces excretion of penicillins. One protocol for Lyme disease gives probenecid with oral ampicillin to attain higher blood levels of the antibiotic; the combination can lead to uric acid stones.

Diagnosis of Uric Acid Stones

Of course, the best way to diagnosis what type of stone a patient has is to have a laboratory analysis using either X-ray crystallography or infra-red spectroscopy. A stone which is visible on sonography but not seen with plain X-ray (a radiolucent stone) has a high probability of being uric acid. If a CT scan has been done, it is useful to have Hounsfield unit counts. A stone in the 300 s is likely to be pure uric acid. A count over 900 indicates the stone is mostly calcium. If the Hounsfield count is between these numbers, the calculus may be of mixed composition.

It is often useful to have the patient measure their urinary pH for three days with narrow range pH paper (e.g. see https://www.microessentiallab.com, item #067). If the urine pH remains below 5.5 most or all of the time during this period, the likelihood that the patient is a uric acid stone former is increased. Some patients only make uric acid stones when they are on ketogenic weight loss diets. In this type of patient, the urinary pH profile may show higher pH values when they are not dieting but will be persistently acid when they are trying to lose weight. Incidentally, the same approach of measuring urinary pH's over a 72-h period may uncover mild renal tubular acidosis in a calcium stone former whose urinary pH does not go below 5.5.

Presentations of Uric Acid Stones

A uric acid stone may present in typical fashion with colic, renal obstruction etc. However, two scenarios are much more common with uric acid than with other calculus minerals. Some patients complain of recurrent lower urinary tract symptoms of urgency, nocturia, and frequency, so-called pseudo-prostatitis. They may be aggravating a mild prostate obstruction with uric acid sludge. Others may have recurrent colic, but no stones are imaged or passed. They may or may not note some gritty material in their urine. This is called the "gravel/colic syndrome." For both of these clinical presentations, the patient whose urine is persistently acid may get relief of symptoms with alkaline salt therapy.

Ureteral Obstruction

The patient with an obstructing stone can often be treated with a stent and then be given alkaline salts to dissolve the stone. Success here depends on free flow of urine past the stone. A calculus in a narrow calyx may not dissolve.

Dissolving and Preventing Uric Acid Stones

1. All stone formers should be encouraged to produce at least 2,000 cc of urine daily. The emphasis should always be on the urine volume and not on just the amount of fluid to be consumed. At high altitudes and in desert climates, insensible fluid losses can be considerable.
2. The diet should try to limit animal protein to 0.8–1.0 g/kg body weight and to minimize other purine sources.
3. Xanthine oxidase inhibitors like allopurinol and febuxostat are indicated for patients with recurrent gout and may be appropriate for hyperuricosuric calcium oxalate stone formers. They are not usually appropriate for the pure uric acid stone former unless alkaline salt therapy fails, as might occur in the setting of bowel disease and diarrhea.
4. Since the solubility of total urate is 11 times greater at pH 6.5 than at pH 5, the effect of controlling urinary acidity is many fold greater than reducing the total urinary urate. Many uric acid stone formers are not hyperuricosuric.

Alkali can be given as a potassium or sodium salt [3]. Advantages of potassium include:

1. Monosodium urate is less soluble than monopotassium urate at higher urinary pH values.
2. Alkaline sodium salts can increase calcium excretion and calcium oxalate crystallization.
3. Large amounts of sodium bicarbonate can increase urinary potassium losses leading to hypokalemia.
4. Many of the patients who form uric acid stones are older or may have hypertension, making it desirable to restrict sodium.

Some pharmacists will mistakenly substitute KCl for K citrate as they are more accustomed to the chloride salt. One source of failure of a treatment regimen can be that the patient has received the wrong preparation.

Sodium bicarbonate is less likely to produce diarrhea, nausea, or a queasy feeling than potassium citrate. It also can be given as a powder bought cheaply in the supermarket.

If the patient has significantly impaired glomerular filtration rate, sodium bicarbonate may be indicated to avoid the risk of hyperkalemia.

Intermittent Versus Continuous Therapy

Alkaline salts can be given two or three times every day to keep the urine pH elevated continuously. Such an approach is usually appropriate if the urinary tract has been stented because one would like to dissolve the stone as quickly as possible. Many physicians simply give 30 mEq alkaline salts TID and do not monitor the urinary pH. I strongly prefer to have the patients check their urinary pHs if for no other reason than to encourage compliance.

If the clinical situation does not make stone dissolution urgent, I only treat the patient once a day [4]. I give 30 mEq potassium citrate plus 30 mEq sodium bicarbonate at one time and have the patient measure the urinary pH 3–4 h later to be sure the pH reaches 7 (see below for available preparations). If the pH does not reach 7.0, I increase the dose until this goal is reached. An occasional patient will be a "slow absorber" and the jump in urinary pH does not occur until after 5–6 h. It may be necessary to ask the patient to re-check the pH at 6 h after dosing if the 3–4 h value is too low. It does not matter what time of day or whether the treatment is taken with meals. When I am trying to dissolve a stone, I have the patient dose every day. When I am just trying to prevent more stones from forming, I give these preparations three times a week. If it takes more than 80 mEq of base to raise the urinary pH, the patient is likely to have substantial lower gastrointestinal fluid losses or to be a protein glutton for whom serious dietary intervention is needed.

The advantages of avoiding continuous therapy are considerable. Alkaline salts can produce diarrhea. In some patients, this effect can be intolerable. However, if the therapy is timed to when the patient is home or near a toilet, the treatment may succeed. Ileostomy patients, and many with other gastrointestinal disorders, can frequently manage these regimens if they take them when they are near a bathroom.

Both sodium and potassium alkaline salts taste bad. Compliance is better if the patient has to take them less often.

Uncontrolled alkaline therapy has the theoretical possibility of causing a shell of hydroxyapatite to form, rendering the stone insoluble. Over treatment can cause a "spaced-out" feeling quite similar to that produced by hyperventilation-induced alkalosis. Hence, intermittent rather than continuous treatment has many advantages but does require the patient to occasionally check the urinary pH to be sure treatment is adequate.

Potassium citrate is available as wax matrix capsules of 10 and 15 mEq. The generic K citrate tablet of 1,080 mg contains 10 mEq. It is often also available in 30 mEq packets of powder which can be dissolved in water. Sodium bicarbonate, baking soda, can be purchased in the supermarket. A flat ½ teaspoon is about 30 mEq. This is a cheap way to medicate but some patients do not like the taste. Sodium bicarbonate also comes in medicinal tables of 650 mg which contain 8 mEq of base. Three K citrate tablets plus four sodium bicarbonate tablets make about 60 mEq of base. Potassium bicarbonate comes as a 25 mEq effervescent tablet that can be dissolved in water and sometimes has better gastrointestinal tolerance for some patients.

As uric acid stones are dissolved, they may become smaller and pass. It is important to warn the patient that it is uncommon but possible that alkaline salt treatment could precipitate colic.

References

1. Shekarriz B, Stoller ML. Uric acid nephrolithiasis: current concepts and controversies. J Urol. 2002;168:1307–14.
2. Maalouf NM, Cameron MA, Moe OW, Adams-Huet B, Sakhaee K. Low urine pH: a novel feature of the metabolic syndrome. Clin J Am Soc Nephrol. 2007;2:883–8.
3. Rodman JS, Williams JJ, Peterson CM. Dissolution of uric acid calculi. J Urol. 1984;131:1039–44.
4. Rodman JS. Prophylaxis of uric acid stones with alternate day doses of alkaline potassium salts. J Urol. 1991;145:97–9.

Part IV
Cystine Stones

Chapter 11
Cystinuria

Michelle A. Baum

Cystinuria is an autosomal recessive disorder of proximal tubular transport of dibasic amino acids—cystine, ornithine, arginine, and lysine (COAL or COLA amino acids). However, only impaired transport of cystine is clinically significant because cystine is poorly soluble in the urine, resulting in recurrent stone formation. In normal individuals, 100 % of filtered cystine is reabsorbed in the proximal tubule.

Cystinuria accounts for approximately 1 % of all stones in adults and 6–10 % in children with the average age of presentation of 12–13 years old [1–4]. Cystinuria results from mutations in one of two components of the proximal tubular cystine transporter system, composed of two subunits linked by a disulfide bridge [5, 6]. The heavy subunit (rBAT) is encoded by gene *SLC3A1* gene on chromosome 2 and the light subunit ($B^{0,+}AT$) is encoded by *SLC7A9* on chromosome 19. $B^{0,+}AT$ is the transporter for neutral (cystine) and dibasic (ornithine, arginine and lysine) amino acids. rBAT modulates trafficking of $B^{0,+}AT$ to the apical membrane of the proximal tubular epithelial cell. Although cystinuria is an autosomal recessive disorder, heterozygote carriers of

M.A. Baum, MD (✉)
Division of Nephrology, Boston Children's Hospital/Harvard Medical School, 300 Longwood Avenue, Boston, MA 02115, USA
e-mail: michelle.baum@childrens.harvard.edu

mutated *SLC7A9* alleles have the pattern of autosomal dominance with incomplete penetrance and have elevated, but not usually clinically significant cystine excretion and rarely form stones.

Prior to the genetic understanding of cystinuria, patients were classified as type I and non-type 1 (type II or III) based on urinary excretion of cystine of their heterozygote parents. Non-type 1 carriers may also have elevated cystine without stone formation. Since the understanding of the genetics of cystinuria, the classification has changed to describe the genetic mutations. Two defective genes for *SLC3A1* result in type A cystinuria and all of these carriers have no detectable cystine in the urine. Two defective genes for *SLC7A9* have Type B cystinuria, and 14 % of heterozygote carriers have no detectable cystine while the remainder have elevated cystine levels but generally do not make stones. One mutated gene in each allele does not cause disease, as two mutations are required of each allele to cause disease. Although very rare (1.6 % of study population in one report), a mutation in one allele of one gene and one allele of the other gene, or more than two mutated alleles (Type AB) can also occur [1, 5, 7]. Although patients now may be classified by their genetic abnormalities in cystinuria, genetic testing is not usually performed as part of day to day clinical care, as there is no difference clinically between the two defects as far as presentation, stone disease, or management. Thus, genetic screening is not routinely performed outside of research protocols.

Clinical suspicion for cystinuria should be high if the patient presents with very large or multiple large stones (staghorn), family history of stones, or refractory recurrent stone disease without a clinical diagnosis. The diagnosis of cystinuria can be made when urinalysis with microscopy demonstrates the classic, pathognomonic hexagonal cystine crystals. Ideally, this should be performed on a first morning urine as it is the most concentrated and will increase the likelihood of observing the crystals. Diagnosis can often be made after a stone analysis following passage of a stone or a procedure. A cyanide-nitroprusside test is also utilized (cyanide reduces cystine to cysteine leading to a color change).

False positives occur in those with other tubular disorders leading to aminoaciduria such as Fanconi syndrome or homocystinuria as well as acetonuria, and patients on certain medications. As previously mentioned, type B heterozygotes (carrier) may also have increased cystine excretion and also a positive cyanide-nitroprusside test. Premature babies and children under age 2 may also have tubular immaturity resulting in increased amino acid excretion and a false positive test [1, 3, 4, 7]. Routine random amino acid analysis can also be sent and will demonstrate elevations in COAL amino acids and random urine cystine to creatinine ratios can be assessed. Ideally, 24-h analysis of cystine excretion should be assessed (commercially available). Normal cystine excretion is 30 mg/day or 0.1 mmol/day (conversion for cystine is 1 mmol=250 mg). These 24-h tests also provide information on 24-h urine volume, pH, citrate excretion as well as cystine supersaturation and a newer measure called cystine capacity, which will be discussed further. These studies are helpful to get baseline characteristics about the patients and to guide initial therapy as well as assess efficacy of therapy [8, 9].

Cystine stones are easily seen on ultrasound. Given that it is a noninvasive test without radiation, ultrasound is the mainstay for evaluation and follow-up. Cystine stones are variably radio-opaque and are not always seen by normal abdominal X-ray. Non-contrast stone protocol CT with low-dose radiation is also helpful to diagnose cystine stones, and also may better characterize size and number.

As with any diagnosis of stone disease, increasing the daily fluid intake is the most important recommendation. However, given the extreme insolubility of cystine in the urine, the recommended fluid requirements of patients with cystinuria must be quite high to maintain high urine output. In adults, fluid intake of a minimum 3–4 L daily is required to decrease the urine cystine concentration to below 250 mg/L to decrease urine supersaturation and stone formation. This includes recommendation for coverage overnight as well, including high fluid intake prior to bedtime and awakening in the middle of the night to drink and void as well. Compliance with high fluid intake is critical to the management of this disorder.

With extremely large fluid intakes, hydration alone could prevent stone recurrence [1, 7, 10].

The second step of cystinuria stone prevention involves increasing the urine pH to above 7 which increases cystine solubility. This is accomplished by using supplementation with citrate or bicarbonate oral preparations. Urine alkalinization with potassium citrate supplementation is preferred over sodium citrate as sodium excretion will increase cystine excretion in the urine. Thus treatment with potassium citrate is also a mainstay of therapy, often three times a day to maintain the pH above 7 [1–4, 7].

Cystine excretion can be reduced by limiting animal protein intake (ingestion of methionine, a cystine precursor). Other effects of lower animal protein intake include decreased renal acid excretion, increasing the urine pH, and reducing the amount of citrate required to alkalinize the urine. Vegetarian diets also reduce renal acid excretion and increase urine pH. However, there have been no randomized controlled studies looking at the effects of dietary protein restriction or vegetarian diet on prevention of cystine stone formation. Thus most patients are advised to maintain the recommended dietary allowance (RDA) for protein required for growth in children and adolescents and approximately 1 g/kg/day in adults. Sodium restriction is also prescribed as high sodium intake results in increased urinary cystine excretion [1, 7].

Lastly, for patients who continue to make stones despite high fluid intake and alkalinization, cystine binding drugs are utilized. D-penicillamine and alpha-mercaptopropionylglycine (tiopronin) break the disulfide bond of cystine and then bind to the sulfhydryl group of the cysteine monomers to make a drug-cysteine complex which is more soluble. Both drugs have significant side effects including changes in taste, rash, neutropenia or thrombocytopenia, abnormal liver function tests, or immune mediated diseases (lupus like or myasthenia gravis like disorders). Furthermore, long-term effects of the cystine binding drugs include membranous nephropathy and thus monitoring for development of proteinuria is important as well. Regular blood tests, at least two to three times yearly, on these medications should include complete blood count, liver function tests, and urine protein assessment. B6 supplementation should be given with penicillamine. Zinc and copper deficiencies may also occur with both medications and levels should also be monitored and supplementation provided where indicated. A usual penicillamine dose is approximately 30 mg/kg/day divided every 6 h, with a maximum dose of 4 g/day. A starting tiopronin dose is 15 mg/kg/day, with an adult dose of 800 mg/day divided two to three times a day. Captopril has also been studied as it has a thiol group but little of it appears in the urine so that results on its reduction of urinary cystine are mixed. Thus, most patients receive either penicillamine or tiopronin therapy when fluids, diet, and alkali do not suffice [1, 7, 9].

Specific 24-h urine collections for cystinuria are very helpful, both in the initial evaluation as well as monitoring for the effects of therapy. If the patient is not receiving treatment with a cystine binding drug, urine volume measurements, pH, and citrate assessment as well as cystine supersaturation values are helpful in following compliance as well as efficacy of fluid intake and alkalinization. With the addition of thiol binding drugs, both measurement of 24-h cystine as well as cystine supersaturation cannot be reliably calculated. Thus, a newer assay was developed called cystine capacity, commercially available in the United States from Litholink Corp (Chicago, IL) [6, 8, 9]. Cystine capacity measures the ability of urine to take up cystine from a preformed solid phase (a result which indicates undersaturation and is a positive value) or release cystine to the solid phase (a result which indicates supersaturation and is a negative value). This measure has been validated to be useful in the presence of cystine binding therapies to aid in monitoring response to the cystine binding drugs as well as other therapies [9]. Thus, the cystine capacity has become a valuable monitoring tool for patients on cystine binding drugs with the goal of achieving a positive value and prescribing the minimally effective doses of cystine binding drugs. With adjustments in medical therapy, or with change in the patient's clinical status with increase in stone formation, as well as at regularly scheduled intervals, 24-h urine collections are critical in assessing efficacy of therapy as well as patient compliance. Frequent visits at a minimum of twice yearly with ultrasound help to determine ongoing metabolic control and occult stone formation as well as reinforce the need for compliance with medications and fluid intake. Patients should be instructed that if they become ill and cannot maintain fluid intake, especially in the face of vomiting or diarrheal illness, they should seek early attention for rehydration to prevent stone formation due to dehydration.

As with other stone disease, surgical treatment of stones greater than 5 mm is usually indicated in cystinuria. However, many clinicians recommend a more aggressive approach to achieve a stone-free state, given that cystine stones can easily and rapidly increase in size and cause morbidity. Treatment by a urologist familiar with cystinuria is important. Extracorporeal shock wave lithotripsy (ESWL) may not be as effective in cystine stone fragmentation compared with calcium stones due to the density of the stone. Ureteroscopy with treatment with holmium laser is very effective. For large stones, percutaneous nephrolithotomy with laser lithotripsy may be indicated. Many large stones may require more than one procedure to achieve a stone-free status [3, 4, 7].

Cystinuria is a complex genetic disorder leading to recurrent stone disease and significant morbidity if not properly managed due to high stone recurrence rates. Given that this disorder presents in childhood and results in a lifelong risk of recurrent nephrolithiasis, treatment of cystinuria may be best managed in a specialty stone clinic with nephrologists familiar with medical management and urologists familiar with surgical management in these complex patients.

References

1. Mattoo A, Goldfarb DS. Cystinuria. Semin Nephrol. 2008;28(2):181–91.
2. Edvardsson V, Goldfarb DS, Lieske J, Beara-Lasic L, Anglani F, Milliner D, Palsson R. Hereditary causes of kidney stones and chronic disease. Pediatr Nephrol. 2013;28:1923–42.

3. Saravakos P, Kokkinou V, Giannotos E. Cystinuria: current diagnosis and management. Urology. 2014;83:693–9.
4. Biyani C, Cartledge J. Cystinuria—diagnosis and management. EAU-EEE Update Series. 2006;4:175–83.
5. Font-Lilijos M, Jimenez-Vidal M, Bisceglia L, Di Perna L, de Sanctis L, Rousaud F, Zelante L, Palacin M, Nunes V. New insights into cystinuria: 40 new mutations, genotype–phenotype correlation, and digenic inheritance causing partial phenotype. J Med Genet. 2005;42:58–68.
6. Sumorok N, Goldfarb DS. Update on cystinuria. Curr Opin Nephrol Hypertens. 2013;22:427–31.
7. Claes D, Jackson E. Cystinuria: mechanisms and management. Pediatr Nephrol. 2012;27:2031–8.
8. Goldfarb DS, Coe F, Asplin J. Urine cystine excretion and capacity in patients with cystinuria. Kidney Int. 2006;69:1041–7.
9. Dolin D, Asplin J, Flagel L, Grasso M, Goldfarb DS. Effect of cystine-binding thiol drugs on urinary cystine capacity in patients with cystinuria. J Endourol. 2005;19(3):429–32.
10. Chillaron J, Font-Llitos M, Fort J, Zorzano A, Goldfarb DS, Nunes V, Palacin M. Pathophysiology and treatment of cystinuria. Nat Rev Nephrol. 2010;6(7):424–34.

Part V
Struvite Stones

Chapter 12
Struvite Stones, Diet and Medications

Ben H. Chew, Ryan Flannigan, and Dirk Lange

General Principles

Struvite stones are a major cause of staghorn calculi. Struvite stones are composed of magnesium, ammonium phosphate. Infection-related stones may also contain calcium carbonate apatite, a crystalline phase of calcium phosphate. They are associated with urinary tract infections with certain bacteria that produce the enzyme urease. Removal of the entire stone is paramount to prevent further stone formation and infections.

Epidemiology

- Struvite stones comprise about 10–15 % of all kidney stones
- They occur more frequently in women in an approximate 2:1 ratio. This is thought to be due to the higher prevalence of urinary tract infections in women.
- Presenting signs are not always typical renal colic as in other stone types, but is usually recurrent urinary tract infections and may include the following with their frequency of occurrence:

B.H. Chew, MD, MSc, FRCSC (✉) • R. Flannigan, MD • D. Lange, MD
Department of Urological Sciences, University of British Columbia,
Level 6 – 2775 Laurel Street, Vancouver, BC, Canada V52 1M9
e-mail: ben.chew@ubc.ca

- 70 % flank/abdominal pain
- 26 % fever
- 18 % gross hematuria
- 8 % asymptomatic
- 1 % sepsis

Risk Factors [1, 2]

- Female gender (2:1 ratio compared to males)
- Extremes of ages
- Congenital urinary tract malformations
- Urinary stasis from obstruction
- Urinary diversion
- Neurogenic bladder (from neurologic disorders including spinal cord injury, spina bifida, multiple sclerosis etc.)
- Chronic indwelling Foley catheters
- Distal renal tubular acidosis
- Medullary sponge kidney
- Diabetes mellitus.

Etiology

- Production of an infection stone requires urea, water, calcium (Ca), magnesium (Mg), phosphate (PO_4), urine with pH>6.8–7.2, and the urease enzyme.
- Bacteria that contain the enzyme, urease, break down urea which results in increasing ammonia and carbon dioxide. Both gram-positive and gram-negative organisms can produce this enzyme.
- Carbonate apatite begins to crystallize at urine pH greater than 6.8 and magnesium ammonium phosphate (struvite) crystallizes at pH greater than 7.2.
- Struvite stones can be found bilaterally in 15 % of cases.
- When the urinary environment is receptive, struvite stones can form rapidly; even within 4–6 weeks [3].

Diagnostic Testing

- Definitive diagnosis is made by stone analysis of magnesium ammonium phosphate or carbonate apatite.
- Microbiological culture of stones is the best source to identify which urease-producing bacteria is responsible, but this is not always detectable. The second best site to identify bacteria is from urine sampled directly from the kidney since it is closest to the site of the infected stone.
- Voided urine culture is not always congruent with the underlying urease-producing bacteria responsible for stone formation.
- The most common species that possess the urease enzyme are *Proteus, Providencia, Serratia ureilytica, and Morganella morganii*. Only 1.4 % of *Escherichia coli* species produce urease.
- If urease-producing bacteria are identified on culture, their mere presence does not always result in struvite stone formation. Despite the fact that up to 39 % of UTIs are associated with urease-producing bacteria, the incidence of struvite stones is still only 16 % suggesting that the presence of a urease positive pathogen is not the only criterion and that other factors must be present in order for a struvite stone to form [3].
- Urine pH is typically greater than 6.8 (>6.8 produces carbonate apatite stones and once >7.2, struvite stones form).

Treatment and Prevention

- As with renal calculi in general, a low sodium diet and high water diet may aid in preventing calculi, as well as modifying risk factors for urinary tract infections such as: limiting foreign bodies to urinary tracts, treating constipation, minimizing stasis of urine, and minimizing immune compromised states. High protein diets have been shown to acidify the urine in veterinary studies and reduce struvite crystals [4], but this is not a proven strategy for struvite stone prevention in humans.

- Treatment and directed therapy of struvite stones is necessary. Conservative non-surgical management however carries a higher 10-year mortality (28 %) compared to those who are managed surgically with stone extraction (7.2 %) [5]. The rate of renal failure is also higher in those managed non-surgically (36 %) compared to those treated with surgery (15.9 %) [1].
- Patients with staghorn calculi who did not undergo surgery were more likely to have renal failure and death (67 %) compared to those who were treated successfully with surgery (0 % mortality) [6]. The same study showed that if infected stone fragments were not entirely cleared, the mortality rate rose from 0 to 2.9 %. Furthermore, the recurrence rate rises to 85 % if residual stone fragments remain.
- Three principles are paramount in the treatment of infection stones [3]:
    - All infected stone burden must be removed
    - Antibiotics must be used to treat the infection to ensure that the urine will be sterile even in the absence of antibiotics.
    - Prevent recurrence by ensuring that both principles 1 and 2 are followed. Subsequent infections must be prevented and all stone must be removed or the cycle will continue.

- There is no set diet to prevent infection stones, and dietary recommendations should be developed and implemented individually, on a case-by-case basis. Acidification therapy with cranberry juice has been used in veterinary studies with some success, but the dosage required would have to be high enough to reduce urine pH [7–9]. Currently, the use of cranberry juice to prevent infection stones remains theoretical in human populations.
    - Acidifying the urine can be helpful in reducing the rate of infection stones, although there is no standardized recommended method [9].
    - Avoiding supplemental magnesium has been shown to be helpful in animal studies [9].
    - Phytonutrients in green tea, turmeric, and berries may reduce the risk of infection [9].

Medications

Antibiotics

- There is very good evidence to utilize antibiotics prior to surgical stone removal as well as following surgery; however, the ideal duration of antibiotic use pre- and post-operatively is widely debated.
- Directed antibiotic therapy aimed at the offending organisms is the preferred therapy. Antibiotics should be administered prior to surgery and for some time following surgery. Complete stone removal is mandatory (see surgical management below) to prevent subsequent infections, sepsis, and stone recurrence.
- Pre-operative oral antibiotics followed by intravenous broad-spectrum antibiotics the day prior to procedure reduce the rates of sepsis. Suppressive antibiotics dosed at ½ frequency should be considered and have been reported in the literature to range from 1 week to 1 year. Antibiotic selection should reflect local antibiograms; however, ciprofloxacin, cefixime, and amoxicillin-clavulanate are three typically sensitive antibiotics to common struvite forming bacteria. Patients should be followed with routine urine cultures and imaged post-operatively to ensure that they remain infection and stone-free. Timing varies by institution, however, both stone and urine cultures should be performed at time of operation, and both imaging and cultures should be repeated within the first 12 weeks post-operatively. Imaging should occur more frequently than with other stone types due to the fact that infection stones may grow very rapidly in the order of 4–6 weeks.

Urease Inhibitors

- Urease inhibitors prevent the enzyme urease from producing further ammonia and carbon dioxide and altering the urine pH, to prevent production of making a favorable

milieu for struvite stones to form. Their use has been shown to provide only a modest benefit.
- The use of *acetohydroxamic acid* has been shown in a randomized double-blind study in patients with chronic urinary tract infections to reduce struvite stone formation from 46 to 17 % [10].
- Side effects of acetohydroxamic acid were quite prevalent in this study thus not favoring the routine clinical use of this therapy. Side effects included dermatological, hematological, and neurological side effects in 22 % of patients treated.

Dissolution Therapy

- Dissolution therapy is a second line treatment for infection stones. Boric acid and permanganate were the first components used for this purpose but are no longer used clinically today.
- *Solution G* was described by Suby in 1944 and is now also known as *Suby's G Solution* [11]. It is an acidic solution (citric acid) that lowers the pH of the urine to dissolve carbonate apatite or struvite crystals.
- *Renacidin R* also alters the urine pH and consists of citric acid, glucono-delta-lactone, and magnesium carbonate [12].
- Use of dissolution therapy is reserved for those patients who are poor surgical candidates as there is a higher risk of mortality from sepsis.
- Rates of success have been reported between 68 and 80 % of cases for dissolution therapy [13, 14].
- Renacidin is no longer FDA approved due to the high rates of sepsis and death.
- Dissolution therapy should be limited to cases where patients would not tolerate surgery. Patients must be admitted to hospital with a nephrostomy tube, Foley catheter, and a normal nephrostogram to ensure that the nephrostomy tube is properly placed with no chance of extravasation. Mean hospital stays of over 30 days are typically required and can be costly to the health care system [15].

Surgery

- The primary therapy for removal of large stone burdens is percutaneous nephrolithotomy (*PCNL*) as recommended by the American Urology Association guideline for staghorn calculi [16]. Shockwave lithotripsy (*SWL*) should not be first-line therapy for large stone burdens, but can be attempted for smaller stone burdens and only if adequate drainage of the kidney is present *prior* to SWL.
    - PCNL is far superior to SWL in a prospective randomized trial. Stone-free rates were 74 % for PCNL compared to 22 % for SWL in a study involving 50 patients with staghorn calculi [17].
- *Ureteroscopy* (*URS*) is a viable *adjunctive* therapy for treating infection stones in combination with PCNL. URS can be used to treat any small fragments that remain after PCNL. URS can be performed in the same sitting as PCNL in an attempt to minimize the number of percutaneous access tracts and has been shown to reduce the amount of blood loss with good stone-free rates [18, 19].
- *Nephrectomy* should be considered in cases where the kidney has negligible function. Kidneys that are damaged from chronic infection and obstruction with severe parenchymal deterioration may act as a source of further infection and if the contralateral kidney is unaffected, nephrectomy is often the best option in these cases [16].
- Open stone surgery (*anatrophic nephrolithotomy*) is rarely necessary in our age of advanced endoscopic techniques, but should be considered if significant anatomical abnormalities exist and if this technique is thought to reduce the number of procedures in order to render the patient stone-free. Obese patients and those with anatomic abnormalities such as infundibular stenosis are potential candidates for this therapy [20]. A randomized trial of open surgery compared to PCNL showed the stone-free rates to be similar, but with many advantages to PCNL including shorter operative times (127 vs 204 min), lower transfusion rate

(14 vs 33 %), shorter hospital stay (6.4 vs 10 days), and earlier return to work (2.5 vs 4.1 weeks) [21].
- Antibiotic therapy pre- and post-operatively is necessary to reduce morbidity and mortality.

Conclusion

- Infection stones occur when bacteria possess the enzyme urease.
- Surgical management and removal of the entire stone is paramount in treatment making PCNL the surgical treatment of choice.
- Antibiotics are another important aspect both prior to and following surgical stone removal. The ideal duration of therapy is unknown. Ensuring a sterile urine environment after stone removal is key to preventing recurrence stones and sepsis.
- Urease inhibitors and dissolution therapy are not routinely recommended and carry a higher rate of sepsis and mortality as well as increased health care costs.

References

1. Koga S, Arakaki Y, Matsuoka M, Ohyama C. Staghorn calculi—long-term results of management. Br J Urol. 1991;68:122–4.
2. Schwartz BF, Stoller ML. Nonsurgical management of infection-related renal calculi. Urol Clin North Am. 1999;26:765–78. viii.
3. Bichler KH, Eipper E, Naber K, Braun V, Zimmermann R, Lahme S. Urinary infection stones. Int J Antimicrob Agents. 2002;19:488–98.
4. Funaba M, Yamate T, Hashida Y, et al. Effects of a high-protein diet versus dietary supplementation with ammonium chloride on struvite crystal formation in urine of clinically normal cats. Am J Vet Res. 2003;64:1059–64.
5. Blandy JP, Singh M. The case for a more aggressive approach to staghorn stones. J Urol. 1976;115:505–6.
6. Teichman JM, Long RD, Hulbert JC. Long-term renal fate and prognosis after staghorn calculus management. J Urol. 1995;153:1403–7.

7. Houston DM, Weese HE, Evason MD, Biourge V, van Hoek I. A diet with a struvite relative supersaturation less than 1 is effective in dissolving struvite stones in vivo. Br J Nutr. 2011;106 Suppl 1:S90–2.
8. Kessler T, Jansen B, Hesse A. Effect of blackcurrant-, cranberry- and plum juice consumption on risk factors associated with kidney stone formation. Eur J Clin Nutr. 2002;56:1020–3.
9. Frassetto L, Kohlstadt I. Treatment and prevention of kidney stones: an update. Am Fam Physician. 2011;84:1234–42.
10. Griffith DP, Gleeson MJ, Lee H, Longuet R, Deman E, Earle N. Randomized, double-blind trial of Lithostat (acetohydroxamic acid) in the palliative treatment of infection-induced urinary calculi. Eur Urol. 1991;20:243–7.
11. Suby HI. Dissolution of urinary calculi. Proc R Soc Med. 1944;37:609–20.
12. Mulvaney WP. The clinical use of renacidin in urinary calcifications. J Urol. 1960;84:206–12.
13. Dretler SP, Pfister RC. Primary dissolution therapy of struvite calculi. J Urol. 1984;131:861–3.
14. Fam B, Rossier AB, Yalla S, Berg S. The role of hemiacidrin in the management of renal stones in spinal cord injury patients. J Urol. 1976;116:696–8.
15. Tiselius H, Hellgren E, Andersson A, Borrud-Ohlsson A, Eriksson I. Minimally invasive treatment of infection staghorn stones with shock wave lithotripsy and chemolysis. Scand J Urol Nephrol. 1999;33:286–90.
16. Preminger GM, Assimos DG, Lingeman JE, et al. Chapter 1: AUA guideline on management of staghorn calculi: diagnosis and treatment recommendations. J Urol. 2005;173:1991–2000.
17. Meretyk S, Gofrit ON, Gafni O, et al. Complete staghorn calculi: random prospective comparison between extracorporeal shock wave lithotripsy monotherapy and combined with percutaneous nephrostolithotomy. J Urol. 1997;157:780–6.
18. Marguet CG, Springhart WP, Tan YH, et al. Simultaneous combined use of flexible ureteroscopy and percutaneous nephrolithotomy to reduce the number of access tracts in the management of complex renal calculi. BJU Int. 2005;96:1097–100.
19. Landman J, Venkatesh R, Lee DI, et al. Combined percutaneous and retrograde approach to staghorn calculi with application of the ureteral access sheath to facilitate percutaneous nephrolithotomy. J Urol. 2003;169:64–7.

20. Assimos D. A comparison of anatrophic nephrolithotomy and percutaneous nephrolithotomy with and without extracorporeal shock wave lithotripsy for management of patients with staghorn calculi. J Urol. 1991;145:710–4.
21. Al-Kohlany KM, Shokeir AA, Mosbah A, et al. Treatment of complete staghorn stones: a prospective randomized comparison of open surgery versus percutaneous nephrolithotomy. J Urol. 2005;173:469–73.

Part VI
Follow-Up of the Recurrent Stone Former

Chapter 13
Laboratory Follow-Up of the Recurrent Stone Former

Sutchin R. Patel

A complete laboratory evaluation is a key component in a recurrent stone former's metabolic work-up. Ensuring that the patient has performed appropriate serum testing along with an analysis of stone composition and a 24-h urine collection is important in helping determine potential etiologies for stone formation and in determining how to best proceed with or adjust dietary and medical interventions. Each of the components in the laboratory evaluation can be important in the follow-up of a recurrent stone former in order to ensure adherence and a response to medical therapy as well as detect any adverse effects of pharmacological treatment. The recent American Urological Association (AUA) Guidelines on the "Medical Management of Kidney Stones" provide a structured and evidence-based approach for the follow-up of the recurrent stone former (Table 13.1).

S.R. Patel, MD (✉)
Department of Urology, University of Wisconsin, School of Medicine and Public Health, 3 S. Greenleaf, Suite J, Gurnee, IL 60031, USA
e-mail: sutchin_patel@yahoo.com

TABLE 13.1. Follow-up—AUA medical management of kidney stones guidelines.

---

1. Clinicians should obtain a single 24-h urine specimen for stone risk factors within 6 months of the initiation of treatment to assess response to dietary and/or medical therapy [*Expert Opinion*]
2. After the initial follow-up, clinicians should obtain a single 24-h urine specimen annually or with greater frequency, depending on stone activity, to assess patient adherence and metabolic response [*Expert Opinion*]
3. Clinicians should obtain periodic blood testing to assess for adverse effects in patients on pharmacological therapy [*Standard*; *Evidence Strength Grade: A*]
4. Clinicians should obtain a repeat stone analysis, when available, especially in patients not responding to treatment [*Expert Opinion*]
5. Clinicians should monitor patients with struvite stones for reinfection with urease-producing organisms and utilize strategies to prevent such occurrences [*Expert Opinion*]
6. Clinicians should periodically obtain follow-up imaging studies to assess for stone growth or new stone formation based on stone activity (plan abdominal imaging, renal ultrasonography, or low dose computed tomography [CT]) [*Expert Opinion*]

Expert Opinion: a statement achieved by consensus of the panel, based on members' clinical training, experience, knowledge, and judgment for which there is no evidence

Standard: a directive statement that an action should or should not be undertaken based on Grade A or Grade B evidence

Recommendation: a directive statement that an action should or should not be undertaken based on Grade C evidence

Grade A Evidence: well-conducted randomized controlled trials or exceptionally strong observational studies

Grade B Evidence: randomized controlled trials with some weaknesses of procedure or generalizability or generally strong observational studies

Grade C Evidence: observational studies that are inconsistent, having small sample size or have other problems that potentially confound interpretation of data

Adapted from Pearle MS, Goldfarb DS, Assimos DG, Curhan G, Denu-Ciocca CJ, Matlaga BR, Monga M, Penniston KL, Preminger GM, Turk TM, White JR. Medical management of kidney stones: AUA guideline. J Urol. 2014;192(2):316–24. With permission from Elsevier

Serum Testing

A basic metabolic panel (including serum glucose, blood urea nitrogen, sodium, potassium, chloride, bicarbonate, creatinine, and calcium) should be obtained in all stone formers.

TABLE 13.2. Adverse effects of medications used to prevent urolithiasis detected via serum testing.

Medication	Effect on serum testing
Thiazide diuretics (HCTZ, chlorthalidone, indapamide)	Hypokalemia, hyperglycemia/glucose intolerance, hyperuricemia, increased serum cholesterol [may also lead to hypocitraturia or hyperuricosuria on urinary testing]
Potassium citrate	Hyperkalemia
Sodium citrate	Hypernatremia
Allopurinol	Elevated LFTs
Tiopronin	Elevated LFTs, Anemia
Acetohydroxamic acid	Anemia

Serum phosphorus and uric acid may also be helpful in the work-up [1, 2]. Serum chemistries may suggest underlying medical conditions associated with stone disease. Hypokalemia and low serum bicarbonate are features of Type 1 renal tubular acidosis. High serum calcium and low serum phosphate would be indicative of primary hyperparathyroidism. Hyperuricemia may suggest a risk of gout [1–3].

A number of medications prescribed for stone prevention are associated with potential adverse effects, some of which can be detected upon follow-up serum testing. Table 13.2 describes common medications used for stone prevention and potential side effects that can be picked up on serum testing. Furthermore thiazide diuretics may uncover patients with primary hyperparathyroidism. Patients with undiagnosed primary hyperparathyroidism may develop hypercalcemia after being started on thiazide therapy [1].

A baseline evaluation of kidney function is necessary and should be tracked over the years that the patient has a history of urolithiasis. Though there has been a correlation between a decrease in glomerular filtration rate and kidney stones, the exact etiology of this association has not been well established and may be multi-factorial (caused by recurrent episodes of ureteral obstruction, repeat urologic interventions, or due to stone disease itself as in the case of nephrocalcinosis) [4].

If serum calcium levels are borderline or elevated (>10.0 mg/dL), measurement of intact parathyroid hormone level is recommended to rule out primary hyperparathyroidism as the etiology of stone formation [1,2]. An ionized serum calcium may be helpful if both serum calcium and PTH are at the high end of the normal values to diagnose primary hyperparathyroidism. Secondary hyperparathyroidism due to vitamin D deficiency would be suspected if PTH is high and serum calcium is low or normal. One would also expect urinary calcium to be low. Measurement of 25-hydroxy-vitamin D would then be indicated (and would be found to be low).

Urinalysis and Stone Analysis

A urinalysis should include both a dipstick and microscopic evaluation to assess urine pH, specific gravity, indicators of infection and to identify crystals pathognomonic of stone type. Assessment of urine pH and specific gravity can also be helpful in monitoring the compliance or efficacy of medical therapy (e.g., potassium citrate) and fluid intake respectively. A urine culture should be obtained in patients with a urinalysis that suggests infection or in patients with recurrent urinary tract infections (UTIs). A high urinary pH (>7.0) or the presence of urea-splitting organisms, such as *Proteus*, *Pseudomonas,* and *Klebsiella*, raises the possibility of struvite stones [3]. Urine pH that is persistently 6.5 or higher, especially in the presence of a low serum bicarbonate concentration suggests distal renal tubular acidosis (RTA). Low urine pH is a frequent cause of uric acid stones.

In recurrent stone formers, available stones should be analyzed by infra-red spectroscopy or X-ray crystallography by a specialty lab to determine their crystalline composition. The presence of uric acid stones could suggest the presence of metabolic syndrome or undiagnosed diabetes. A predominant hydroxyapatite component, or less frequently, brushite (both forms of calcium phosphate), in a stone can be seen in the case of renal tubular acidosis or primary hyperparathyroidism and would warrant an assessment of serum bicarbonate, calcium,

13. Laboratory Follow-Up of the Recurrent Stone Former

and phosphorus. The finding of a struvite or magnesium ammonium phosphate stone would suggest an infectious etiology. Patients with struvite stones may be at risk for continued recurrent urinary tract infections and thus should be monitored to make sure their infections, and more importantly, the source of their infections are completely treated. Pure calcium oxalate stones or stones with mixed composition may be less useful in determining a diagnostic etiology as they may occur in several entities.

Crystals noted on microscopy of urine sediment may help identify the type of stone formed if a stone analysis has not been performed on an extracted or passed stone [3] (Fig. 13.1). Hexagonal crystals confirm cystinuria. Coffin-lid shaped crystals are pathognomonic for magnesium ammonium phosphate (struvite) crystals which are associated with urea-splitting organisms such as *Proteus mirabilis*. Calcium oxalate monohydrate crystals are dumbbell-shaped, while calcium oxalate dihydrate crystals are shaped like envelopes (tetrahedral, bipyramidal crystals). Brushite crystals are often needle shaped. Uric acid crystals can vary in shape from amorphous shards or plates to rhomboids or needles. Amorphous crystals are called urates if urine pH is 5, and phosphates if urine pH is 6.5 or higher. Urinary crystals can also be found in patients taking certain medications. For example sulfadiazine and sulfamethoxazole crystals appear as "shocks of wheat."

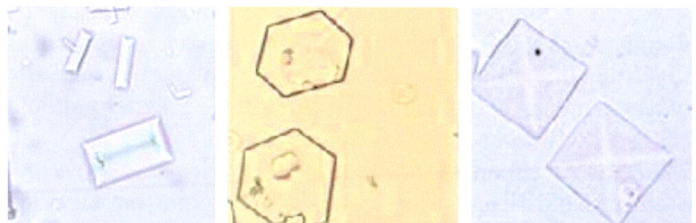

FIG. 13.1. Urinary crystals noted on microscopy. *Left*: struvite (coffin-lid), *Center*: cystine (hexagonal), *Right*: calcium oxalate dihydrate (envelope, tetrahedral)

The AUA Guidelines for the "Medical Management of Kidney Stones" state that clinicians should obtain a repeat stone analysis when available and especially in patients not responding to therapy [1]. Changes in stone composition have been reported in calcium oxalate stone formers who have converted to forming calcium phosphate stones. Uric acid stone formers and some cystine stone formers may also have additional metabolic abnormalities that predispose them to form other stones.

24-Hour Urine Collection

A 24-h urine collection should be recommended in "high risk" or recurrent stone formers [1–3]. "High risk" stone formers include those with a family history of stone disease, recurrent urinary tract infections, pediatric stone formers, obesity, malabsorptive intestinal disease, history of gastric bypass surgery, solitary kidney (because of the serious implications of ureteral obstruction in a patient with a solitary kidney), other medical conditions that can predispose to stone formation (such as primary hyperparathyroidism, gout, diabetes mellitus type 2, renal tubular acidosis type 1). Recurrent stone formers include those patients with repeat stone episodes as well as those patients with multiple stones at first presentation. Interested first-time stone formers may also be offered metabolic testing to help prevent the risk of future stone recurrence.

Either 1 or 2 separate 24-h urine collections may be obtained, as there is controversy and no clear consensus regarding the accuracy of a single collection and the necessity of a second urine collection [1, 2, 5, 6]. The patient should choose a day when all voids can be collected completely and when the specimen would represent a "typical day." The first morning void is discarded and from that point on, all urine must be collected in the appropriate laboratory-provided container. When the patient wakes up the following morning, the first morning void is collected with the rest of the specimen.

Prior to analyzing a patient's 24-h urine results one must determine the adequacy of the specimen collection [3]. Total urinary creatinine is measured as an internal check (males: 15–20 mg of creatinine per kg of body weight in 24 h; females: 10–15 mg of creatinine per kg of body weight in 24 h) [3]. Total 24-h urinary creatinine values for the patient that are abnormal may be due to under/over collection or if the patient has greater than or less than the expected muscle mass. After checking to make sure that the patient performed a collection correctly, if there is any question about the adequacy of the specimen, one should consider a repeat 24-h urine collection. A number of commercially available 24-h urine analysis kits are available. It is important to note that the "normal limits" cited on each kit may not be the same between different companies.

Urine supersaturation of stone forming salts has been shown to correlate with stone composition. Supersaturation, calculated using the EQUIL2 formula, is reported in most commercially available 24-h urine collection results. The saturation index (as calculated using the JESS computer program) is commercially reported and has been found to provide a more reliable estimation of urinary saturation than the EQUIL2. Because a calculated supersaturation index takes into account multiple urinary variables, it can be helpful in predicting stone risk and can be used to guide and monitor the effectiveness of treatment [2, 7, 8]. Careful attention should be paid to the urine pH of the 24-h urine collection as uric acid can precipitate at a low pH thus leading to an inaccurate urinary uric acid measurement (underestimation). Thus it is important to make sure that the urine sample was alkalinized in order to allow the uric acid to be fully dissolved and thus get an accurate urinary uric acid measurement.

A repeat 24-h urine collection should be obtained within 6 months after the initiation of dietary or medical interventions in order to judge the efficacy of the treatment and to provide patients with feedback [1]. It is important not to use 24-h urinary parameters as surrogates for an assessment of the patient's habitual diet. Certain renal excretory components are under tight homeostatic control, such as calcium, and are not necessarily reflective of intake. Other urinary parameters have endogenous contributors, such as uric acid and oxalate, and may therefore not always be linked with diet. Dietary assessment can help to corroborate findings in the 24-h urine collection and can rule "in" or "out" diet as contributory to specific urinary derangements. Markers of protein intake such as urinary uric acid or urinary sulfate may be reflective of protein intake and can be used to assess dietary modifications or adherence to treatment. Likewise, urinary potassium when compared to a baseline measurement can be used to gauge adherence to medication regimens such as potassium citrate. In patients with known cystine stones or a family history of cystinuria, urinary cystine should be measured. In patients with recurrent cystine urolithiasis, urinary cystine can serve as a surrogate marker for the effectiveness of the patient's current therapy (total urine volume, urinary citrate, and urine pH are generally also followed). Use of the oral and fasting calcium load test to distinguish among the types of hypercalciuria is not recommended as it has not been shown to change clinical practice [1]. Once a patient's urinary parameters are stable or have been optimized, a single 24-h urine specimen should be obtained annually or with greater frequency depending on whether the patient has a stone recurrence [1].

References

1. Pearle MS, Goldfarb DS, Assimos DG, Curhan G, Denu-Ciocca CJ, Matlaga BR, Monga M, Penniston KL, Preminger GM, Turk TM, White JR. Medical management of kidney stones: AUA guideline. J Urol. 2014;192(2):316–24.
2. Goldfarb DS, Arowojolu O. Metabolic evaluation of first-time and recurrent stone formers. Urol Clin North Am. 2013;40:13–20.
3. Ferrandino MN, Pietrow PK, Preminger GM. Evaluation and medical management of urinary lithiasis. In: Wein AJ, Kavoussi LR, Novick AC, Partin AW, Peters CA, editors. Campbell-Walsh urology. 10th ed. Philadelphia: Saunders Elsevier; 2012.
4. Rule AD, Bergstralh EJ, Melton III LJ, et al. Kidney stones and the risk for chronic kidney disease. Clin J Am Soc Nephrol. 2009;4:804–11.

5. Pak CY, Peterson R. Adequacy of a single stone risk analysis in the medical evaluation of urolithiasis. J Urol. 2001;165:378–81.
6. Parks JH, Goldfisher E, Asplin J, et al. A single 24-hour urine collection is inadequate for the medical evaluation of nephrolithiasis. J Urol. 2002;167:1607–12.
7. Pearle MS, Lotan Y. Etiology, epidemiology, and pathogenesis. In: Wein AJ, Kavoussi LR, Novick AC, Partin AW, Peters CA, editors. Campbell-Walsh urology. 10th ed. Philadelphia: Saunders Elsevier; 2012.
8. Parks JH, Coward M, Coe FL. Correspondence between stone composition and urine supersaturation in nephrolithiasis. Kidney Int. 1997;51:894–900.

Chapter 14
Imaging (Cost, Radiation)

Michael E. Lipkin

Imaging is an important component in the evaluation of the recurrent stone former. The American Urological Association Guidelines for the Medical Management of Kidney Stones recommend periodic imaging to assess for stone activity [1]. The guidelines state that stable patients should be imaged on a yearly basis. The choice of imaging study is based on a number of factors. These include patient and stone characteristics. Patient characteristics that are important to consider include body habitus and age. One of the most important stone characteristic that factors into deciding on the appropriate imaging study is whether or not the stone is radio-opaque.

Radiation exposure and cost of imaging studies play a large role in determining the appropriate study to use to follow recurrent stone formers. Patients with nephrolithiasis are at risk for significant radiation exposure from both diagnostic imaging and fluoroscopy used during treatment. Every effort should be made to minimize the amount of radiation these patients are exposed to. In addition to reducing radiation exposure, cost is an important consideration when choosing an

M.E. Lipkin, MD (✉)
Division of Urology, Surgery, Duke University Medical Center,
40 Duke Medicine Circle, DUMC 3167, Durham, NC 27710, USA
e-mail: Michael.lipkin@duke.edu

imaging study to follow a recurrent stone former. All of the above factors must be balanced when deciding on the most appropriate imaging study to follow these patients.

Non-contrast Computed Tomography

Non-contrast computed tomography of the abdomen and pelvis (NCCT) is considered the gold standard imaging for the evaluation of patients with nephrolithiasis. This is particularly true for patients with flank pain and suspected ureteral stones. The sensitivity and specificity for NCCT for the detection of urolithiasis has been reported to be 95–98 % and 96–98 %, respectively [2].

The main drawbacks of NCCT in the follow-up of recurrent stone formers are the significant amount of radiation it exposes patients to and the cost. The reported effective dose for a standard NCCT of the abdomen and pelvis is between 8 and 16 mSv [3]. Recent improvements in CT scanners and software have allowed for a significant reduction in the dose from NCCT. Though there is no strict definition of low dose NCCT, in general any NCCT performed for the evaluation of urolithiasis with an effective dose ≤3 mSv is considered low dose [3]. A recent meta-analysis evaluating the performance of low dose NCCT compared to standard dose NCCT found a pooled sensitivity of 97 % and specificity of 95 % for low dose NCCT [3].

Despite the excellent sensitivity of low dose NCCT, there are some limitations for its use in the follow-up of stone formers. It has reduced sensitivity in obese patients. In a study comparing low dose to standard dose NCCT for the evaluation of patients with renal colic, the sensitivity of low dose NCCT was found to be decreased in patients with a body mass index (BMI) ≥ 30 kg/m^2 [4]. When specifically evaluating renal calculi, the sensitivity of low dose NCCT was reduced for stones < 3 mm in patients with a BMI ≥ 30 kg/m^2 versus those with a BMI < 30 kg/m^2 (33 versus 63 %, respectively).

Although low dose NCCT has less radiation exposure than a standard NCCT, it still exposes patients to more radiation than a plain abdominal radiography (0.5 mSv) or digital tomosynthesis (0.85 mSv) [5]. It also has more radiation than a renal ultrasound (RUS) which has no radiation. There have been reports of ultra-low-dose NCCT which have an effective dose similar to a plain abdominal radiograph (KUB) [6]. The possible role of ultra-low-dose NCCT for evaluation of the recurrent stone former is currently unclear.

Another issue for standard NCCT, low dose NCCT, and ultra-low-dose NCCT for the follow-up of the recurrent stone former is cost. The cost will vary institution from institution and country to country. At our institution, the total cost of a NCCT of the abdomen and pelvis is more than 10× that of a KUB and 5× that of a RUS. In general, the use of CT should play a limited role for the routine follow-up of the recurrent stone former. It is indicated in the recurrent stone former with flank pain and can be considered in patients with radio-lucent stones in whom it is critical to know their stone burden.

Renal Ultrasound

Renal ultrasound (RUS) is routinely indicated in the follow-up of patients with ureteral stones who have undergone surgical management [7]. Its use for the routine follow-up of recurrent stone formers is less clear. The reported sensitivities and specificities of RUS for the detection of renal stones vary greatly [2]. The sensitivity of RUS for the detection of renal calculi has been reported to be 29–81 % and the specificity has been reported to be 82–90 %. Another limitation of RUS for the follow-up of recurrent stone formers is the tendency to over-estimate stone size [8]. In one study, RUS over-estimated stone size by approximately 2 mm when compared to NCCT [8]. The discordance in stone size worsened as skin to stone distance increased. It is also more difficult for RUS to detect stones in patients who are obese.

Despite these limitations, there are a number of advantages in using RUS for the follow-up of recurrent stone formers. Ultrasound does not utilize any radiation, thus making it the ideal study in the pediatric population and in pregnant women. It can detect secondary signs of obstruction such as hydronephrosis, which can be important in the recurrent stone former who complains of intermittent flank pain. The cost of a RUS is significantly less than a NCCT. At our institution, a RUS is about 5× less expensive than a NCCT. In patients at risk for calcium based stones and uric acid stones, such as those with gouty diathesis, RUS in combination with KUB may be the ideal follow-up imaging study. This minimizes radiation exposure when compared to NCCT or low dose NCCT. The cumulative cost of a RUS and KUB is still significantly less than NCCT.

Plain Abdominal Radiography

Plain abdominal radiography (KUB) has historically been the imaging modality of choice for the evaluation of patients with nephrolithiasis. This is due to the fact that the majority of stones are calcium based and therefore expected to be visible on KUB. The sensitivity and specificity of KUB for the detection of nephrolithiasis has been reported to be between 45–58 % and 69–77 % [2]. Despite the relatively low sensitivity and specificity, if a stone is radio-opaque and visible on KUB it is an ideal study to follow a recurrent stone former. Compared to other imaging modalities such as US and NCCT, KUB is inexpensive. The radiation dose from a KUB has been reported to be 0.5 mSv, which is lower than the dose of a NCCT or a low dose NCCT [5]. Other advantages of KUB for the follow-up of the recurrent stone former are that it can be quickly performed and is often available in a physician's office.

The disadvantages for KUB in the follow-up of stone formers include the inability to image radio-lucent stones such as uric acid stones. In addition, overlying bowel gas can often obscure the visualization of stones. It is also not able to detect signs of obstruction, which is important for patients who report flank pain. It may be difficult to detect very small stones in the kidney on KUB, as well.

KUB with Tomograms

Tomographic images are captured by performing a sweeping arc with the X-ray emitter. The arc is focused on a specific depth. Images can be taken at multiple depths, with the resolution of the image optimized at the assigned depth. In a study comparing the detection or renal stones in 127 consecutive patients, tomograms detected additional stones compared to KUB in 37 % of the cases [9].

Despite the increased detection of stones, KUB with tomograms are not commonly performed anymore. They have largely been supplanted by NCCT. Compared to plain KUB, KUB and tomograms are more costly. The amount of radiation from KUB with tomograms is largely dependent on how many tomographic images. One study demonstrated that for each tomographic sweep, patients are exposed to 1.1 mSv [10]. Assuming three tomographic sweeps, the cumulative effective dose from KUB and tomograms would be 3.93 mSv. This is greater than the exposure from either a KUB or a low dose NCCT. In general, KUB and tomograms are of limited utility in the follow-up of recurrent stone formers.

Digital Tomosynthesis

Digital tomosynthesis (DT) is a new technology derived from KUB and tomograms. In DT, a single tomographic sweep is performed after a scout KUB. A digital flat panel detector records all of the data from the sweep and software reconstructs the data into a number of coronal slice images. The coronal images are each focused at a different depth. In each slice, overlying structures are removed and only the structures at that depth are in focus.

Digital tomosynthesis has been shown to have improved sensitivity for detecting stones in the kidney [5]. Using NCCT as the standard reference, DT has been shown to have a sensitivity of 66 % for the detection of stones in the kidney compared to 24 % for KUB. In addition, DT was more sensitive at detecting smaller stones. The sensitivities for detecting stones ≤2 mm, 2–5 mm, and >5 mm for DT were 36, 64, and 76 %, respectively. In comparison, the sensitivities of KUB for the same stone size groupings were 3, 28, and 54 %, respectively [5]. The radiation exposure from DT is slightly greater than a single KUB, but less than that of a low dose NCCT. The reported effective dose for DT is 0.85 mSv, compared to 0.5 mSv for KUB and approximately 3 mSv for most low dose CT [3, 5]. It is difficult to determine the costs of DT as it is a new technology. At our institution, the cost is the same as KUB and tomograms which is double the cost of a KUB, but less costly than RUS or NCCT. There is also a capital investment for DT since it requires a digital panel detector.

Conclusion

The ideal imaging study for the follow-up of recurrent stone formers would have a high sensitivity for the detection of stones, minimal or no radiation exposure, and would be low cost. Unfortunately, this combination of factors does not exist in any current imaging modality (Table 14.1). The choice of imaging study as well as the interval between imaging for follow-up of the recurrent stone former must be made balancing these variables with clinical factors such as stone composition, body habitus, risk of obstruction, and need for accuracy (Fig. 14.1). In general, for patients whose stones are visible on KUB, KUB is an excellent imaging modality for follow-up. For those with radio-lucent stones, either RUS or NCCT should be utilized. Digital tomosynthesis holds promise for the future follow-up of recurrent stone formers, however more studies need to be performed to determine the diagnostic accuracy across a range of stone compositions and body sizes.

TABLE 14.1. Comparison of different imaging modalities for the follow-up of the recurrent stone former.

	Diagnostic accuracy	Radiation exposure	Cost
Non-contrast computed tomography	++++	+	+
Low dose NCCT	+++	++	+
Ultrasound	++	++++	++
Plain abdominal radiography (KUB)	+	+++	++++
KUB with tomograms	++	+	+++
Digital tomosynthesis	++	+++	+++

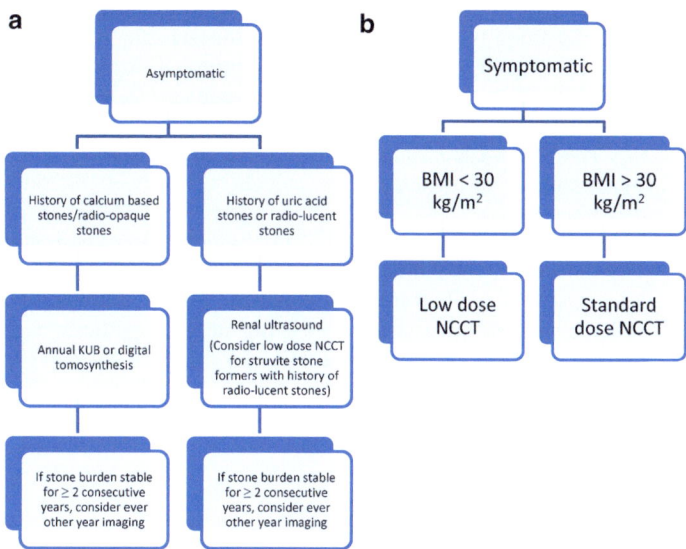

FIG. 14.1. Imaging of the recurrent stone former. (**a**) imaging for the asymptomatic patient (**b**) imaging for the symptomatic patient

References

1. Pearle MS, et al. Medical management of kidney stones: AUA guideline. J Urol. 2014;192(2):316–24.
2. Lipkin ME, Preminger GM. Imaging techniques for stone disease and methods for reducing radiation exposure. Urol Clin North Am. 2013;40(1):47–57.

3. Niemann T, Kollmann T, Bongartz G. Diagnostic performance of low-dose CT for the detection of urolithiasis: a meta-analysis. AJR Am J Roentgenol. 2008;191(2):396–401.
4. Poletti PA, et al. Low-dose versus standard-dose CT protocol in patients with clinically suspected renal colic. AJR Am J Roentgenol. 2007;188(4):927–33.
5. Mermuys K, et al. Digital tomosynthesis in the detection of urolithiasis: diagnostic performance and dosimetry compared with digital radiography with MDCT as the reference standard. AJR Am J Roentgenol. 2010;195(1):161–7.
6. Kluner C, et al. Does ultra-low-dose CT with a radiation dose equivalent to that of KUB suffice to detect renal and ureteral calculi? J Comput Assist Tomogr. 2006;30(1):44–50.
7. Fulgham PF, et al. Clinical effectiveness protocols for imaging in the management of ureteral calculus disease: AUA technology assessment. J Urol. 2013;189(4):1203–13.
8. Ray AA, et al. Limitations to ultrasound in the detection and measurement of urinary tract calculi. Urology. 2010;76(2):295–300.
9. Goldwasser B, et al. Role of linear tomography in evaluation of patients with nephrolithiasis. Urology. 1989;33(3):253–6.
10. Astroza GM, et al. Radiation exposure in the follow-up of patients with urolithiasis comparing digital tomosynthesis, non-contrast CT, standard KUB, and IVU. J Endourol. 2013;27(10):1187–91.

Chapter 15
What to Do About Asymptomatic Calculi

Shubha De and Sri Sivalingam

Primary Asymptomatic Stones

Asymptomatic stones can take many forms. Those causing silent obstruction require immediate attention and will not be considered here. Non-obstructing renal stones lacking discernable signs and symptoms will also be considered separately from post-therapeutic *residual fragments* in this chapter.

Though overall rates are unknown, routinely screened cohorts (i.e., colon cancer, living kidney donors) have shown rates of 7–9.8 % of incidental stones on CT imaging. In those with incidental stones, 13.5 % had a pre-existing diagnosis of kidney stones. Subsequent stone related events were experienced by 45 % of those with incidental stones, 1.3 ± 1.1 years after their initial imaging.

The natural history of asymptomatic stones has been described by six studies [1–6]. Five studies retrospectively assessed those who were diagnosed with incidental stones, and attempted to characterize the risk factors for subsequent stone related events (pain, spontaneous passage, surgical intervention, or increase in size). Ranging from 50 to 340

S. De, MD, FRCPC (✉) • S. Sivalingam, MD, MSC, FRCSC
Cleveland Clinic, Glickman Urological and Kidney Institute,
10510 Park Lane, Cleveland, OH 44106, USA
e-mail: shubhade@gmail.com

patients, follow-up over 3–4 years identified 30–70 % of patients eventually developed symptoms, a third of whom required emergency room attention. However, over half of all patients who develop symptoms appear to pass their stones spontaneously, and only 12–35 % go on to require surgical intervention. Kaplan Meyer curves estimate the 5-year risk of developing future symptoms as 45–48 % [2, 4].

Pelvic, followed by upper pole locations are most likely to progress to symptomatic stones. Larger stones (>15 mm), in addition to a history of multiple stones and recurrent stone disease have also been shown to increase the rates of progression to symptoms. Data from prospectively followed patients show lower pole stones may increase in size more readily than other locations, though they tend to have lower rates of stone related events, and require intervention less often (10 % at 4 years) than other locations. In terms of urinary indices, one study found stone growth is linked to hyperuricosuria, though stone composition was not be shown to affect growth kinetics [2].

Residual Fragments

Fragments left after surgical intervention appear to have a divergent natural history. Though conceptually similar, several studies have described their unique clinical course after various lithotripsy modalities. After SWL, residual fragments ≤4 mm have been prospectively shown to result in symptomatic episodes or require intervention in 70 % of patients by 5 years. This is notably higher than 5-year estimates of progression (to stone related events) in primary asymptomatic stones. After PCNL, 70 % of patients with fragments >2 mm develop a stone related event, whereas even fragments ≤2 mm cause symptoms or require medical attention in 43 % of patients. Though the 5-year probability of a fragment related event is 48 % and similar to incidental stones, significantly higher rates of secondary procedures (up to 53 %) are required for patients with known residual stones.

Follow-Up

No consensus exists as to how these patients should be followed once observation is deemed appropriate. In reviewing published study designs and practice patterns, follow-up strategies range in frequency (3–12 months), utilization of imaging modalities (X-ray, IVP, ultrasound, low dose CT), and the inclusion of lab tests (serum creatinine, urinalysis, and/or urine cultures). With increasing concerns of the over radiation exposure and medical costs, X-ray (± ultrasound) tends to be adequate in most patients with longer durations (i.e., 12 months) suggested in stable disease.

Treatment

In dealing with silent obstruction, or asymptomatic staghorn calculi, treatment is clearly indicated. However, for smaller non-obstructing stones which have no causing issues, intervention is presupposed on the notion of preventing future acute episodes, or treating while stones are amenable to less morbid procedures.

Urologists often consider stone size, position, and Hounsfield units to guide decision-making. Since smaller stones (≤4 mm) are most amenable to passage, these are most often observed. This is highlighted by a survey of over 160 American urologist, where 90 % reported preferentially observing stones <5 mm. However only 25 % would observe stones >5 mm, whereas 60 % would recommend SWL. Similarly, when patients were presented with a hypothetical 8 mm lower pole stone, 22 % chose observation, while 48 % chose SWL. Their preferred therapeutic modality was strongly influenced by their stone burden and previous interventions.

One prospective randomized study assessed SWL versus observation in patients with asymptomatic stones <15 mm, with a mean follow-up of 26 months. SWL reduced patients' stone burdens, though no overall differences were seen in quality of life or renal function. In the observational arm only

9 % required intervention, calling into question the role of SWL for this group [7]. A subgroup analysis from a retrospective study identified a small number of patients with stones >15 mm, almost all of whom developed stone related events requiring intervention [2]. Another study investigating stones, lower pole stones <20 mm randomized patients to observation, SWL, and PCNL. PCNL was superior to SWL for stone clearance, at the expense of increased morbidity [8]. At a median of 22 months, approximately 20 % of observed patients required intervention.

As such, it can be seen that the 2-year risk of intervention increases with stone size, though lower pole stones can be observed with less risk. As two retrospective studies documented 43–45 % of all asymptomatic stones reside in the lower pole, PCNL is considered the most efficacious for these stones >10 mm, whereas ureteroscopy has been found equivalent to SWL in lower pole stones <10 mm (as of 2003).

Pelvic and upper pole stones, in addition to those with recurrent or multiple stones are more likely to cause symptoms. As such these patients must be counseled appropriately if undergoing observation. However, they can be reassured that of those that develop symptoms only a small number require surgery.

Selective medical therapy has been shown to reduce the post procedural (PCNL and SWL) stone formation and recurrence rate, in those with or without residual fragments [9]. Similar findings have been reported in recurrent stone formers, who additionally benefitted from a significant reduction in necessary surgical procedures. Dissolution therapy can also be employed for known uric acid stone formers, mitigating the need for surgery all together.

Special Groups

Specific cohorts may benefit from the prophylactic intervention when an acute event could lead to catastrophic results. Frail patients, and those with significant medical comorbidities, who cannot tolerate physiologic stressors of pain (i.e., severe coronary artery disease), fluid shifts (i.e., congestive heart failure), and long periods of immobility (i.e., Multiple Sclerosis) might be considered for up front, definitive management. Those with solitary kidneys (± transplant grafts), or chronic renal dysfunction should be monitored closely or considered for early intervention as transient obstruction may lead to acute renal injury or further renal impairment. Anatomic abnormalities precluding spontaneous passage and complicating intervention (i.e., UPJO, ureteric strictures, ureteric re-implantation) should be considered early, with a goal of complete stone removal.

Populations predisposed to infections and stones (i.e., spinal cord injury, Spina bifida, neurogenic bladder), will need careful consideration and management of both. In addition, improved bladder management strategies will often be required to reduce future risks.

Social factors such as employment type, travel schedule, and responsibilities should also be investigated, as many patients cannot afford the down time associated with unexpected medical issues. Prospective quality of life assessments of stone formers (asymptomatic + symptomatic) using the NIH PROMIS QoL survey identified primary care givers (i.e., parents), those with chronic medical comorbidities, or recurrent stone disease to have worsened QoL scores. This suggests that these patients may benefit from more timely stone management, and it is important to consider social and financial responsibilities, in addition to health related issues.

Conclusion

Approximately half of all patients with asymptomatic stones will progress to having symptoms within 5 years. A third of those patients will need emergency room attention, however only half will require surgical intervention. Lower pole stones tend to represent the majority of asymptomatic stones and are least likely to progress to symptomatic events or require surgical intervention. Whereas residual fragments have a much higher risk of requiring subsequent procedures.

In predicting who will eventually have a stone related event, stone location (renal pelvis and upper pole), size (>15 mm), and a history of recurrent or multiple stones may increase one's risk. Special consideration should be given to patients' medical history and social/financial responsibilities, in attempts to minimize the burden of disease.

References

1. Glowacki LS, Beecroft ML, Cook RJ, Pahl D, Churchill DN. The natural history of asymptomatic urolithiasis. J Urol. 1992;147:319–21.
2. Burgher A, Beman M, Holtzman JL, Monga M. Progression of nephrolithiasis: long-term outcomes with observation of asymptomatic calculi. J Endourol. 2004;18:534–9.
3. Goyal NK, Goel A, Sankhwar S. Outcomes of long-term follow-up of patients with conservative management of asymptomatic renal calculi. BJU Int. 2012;110:E5–6.
4. Kang HW, Lee SK, Kim WT, Kim Y-JJ, Yun S-JJ, Lee S-CC, et al. Natural history of asymptomatic renal stones and prediction of stone related events. J Urol. 2013;189:1740–6.
5. Koh L-TT, Ng F-CC, Ng K-KK. Outcomes of long-term follow-up of patients with conservative management of asymptomatic renal calculi. BJU Int. 2012;109:622–5.
6. Inci K, Sahin A, Islamoglu E, Eren MT, Bakkaloglu M, Ozen H. Prospective long-term followup of patients with asymptomatic lower pole caliceal stones. J Urol. 2007;177:2189–92.
7. Keeley FX, Tilling K, Elves A, Menezes P, Wills M, Rao N, et al. Preliminary results of a randomized controlled trial of prophylactic shock wave lithotripsy for small asymptomatic renal calyceal stones. BJU Int. 2001;87:1–8.
8. Yuruk E, Binbay M, Sari E, Akman T, Altinyay E, Baykal M, et al. A prospective, randomized trial of management for asymptomatic lower pole calculi. J Urol. 2010;183:1424–8.
9. Kang DE, Maloney MM, Haleblian GE, Springhart WP, Honeycutt EF, Eisenstein EL, et al. Effect of medical management on recurrent stone formation following percutaneous nephrolithotomy. J Urol. 2007;177:1785–8. discussion 1788–9.

Part VII
Managing Recurrence

Chapter 16
Acute Renal Colic and Medical Expulsive Therapy

Charles D. Scales Jr. and Eugene G. Cone

Acute Renal Colic

Defined as a combination of the following: pain of short (≤12 h) duration, nausea/vomiting, flank pain, anorexia, and/or hematuria (≥10,000/mm^3 erythrocytes on urinalysis) [1].

Differential Diagnosis

- *Renal or ureteral stone*
- *Acute uncomplicated pyelonephritis*

    - Signs and symptoms can be extremely similar
    - If fever ≥38 °C, imaging is mandatory to rule out obstruction

- *Renal infarction* and/or *renal vein thrombosis*

    - Have a higher degree of suspicion in patients at increased risk or with a history of thromboembolic disease

---

C.D. Scales Jr., MD, MSHS (✉) • E.G. Cone, MD
Division of Urologic Surgery, Duke University Medical Center,
40 Duke Medicine Circle, Suite 1570, White Zone,
Durham, NC 27710, USA
e-mail: chuck.scales@duke.edu

- *Uretero-pelvic junction obstruction*
  - Especially after high volume fluid intake, which increases urine output and can dilate the pelvis causing obstructive pain
- *Testicular torsion* and/or *torsion of the appendix testis*
  - Most common in children and early adolescent males
- *Spontaneous renal hemorrhage*
  - Can be caused by kidney masses (including angiomyolipoma), bleeding diathesis, or occult trauma
- *Renal papillary necrosis*
  - More common in systemic disease including diabetes mellitus, sickle cell crisis, and analgesic nephropathy
  - Pain is caused as sloughed papillae obstruct the ureter

Lab work

- *Complete blood cell count* (white cells, red cells, and platelets)
- *Blood chemistry* (creatinine, uric acid, sodium, potassium, ionized calcium)
- *Urinalysis* (including red and white cells, bacteria, nitrite, approximate pH)
- If febrile additional testing is warranted
  - *C Reactive Protein*

    EAU guidelines recommend obtaining CRP in febrile patients to help determine the need for diversion or stent placement. CRP > 28 better predicts a need for urinary diversion than even a leukocytosis or elevation of serum creatinine value [2]

  - *Urine Culture*
  - *Coagulation studies* (PT/INR and PTT)

Imaging

Patients presenting with flank pain, fever, and a suspected stone should receive prompt imaging. This is particularly true of patients with solitary kidney, and of patients in whom the diagnosis is unclear and imaging would be of assistance.

Non-contrast enhanced computed tomography (NCCT) is the imaging modality of choice to confirm stone diagnosis in patients with acute flank pain [3, 4].

- Patients with a BMI of ≤30 should be considered for low-dose NCCT
- Digitally enhanced CT is preferred because it allows for 3D reconstruction of the collecting system, as well as easy calculation of skin-to-stone distance and stone density, two important predictors of procedural success rates
- NCCT has a sensitivity and specificity of 94–100 %
- NCCT also has the benefit of elucidating non-urinary pathology in about 1/3 of patients who present with acute flank pain

Supportive Therapy

Initial therapy is aimed at supporting the patient, and consists of *analgesia* and *hydration*

Analgesia

Pain relief should be initiated immediately

NSAIDs should be looked to as first-line therapy whenever possible [5].

- *Diclofenac sodium* 75 mg IV bolus or 100–150 mg Extended Release PO/PR QD
  - Diclofenac has no effect on renal function in patients with a normal glomerular filtration rate (GFR), but can affect renal function in those with a pre-existing decrease in their GFT

– Specifically recommended by EAU guidelines to reduce recurrent colic
- *Ketorolac* 30 mg IV slow infusion QID (can also be administered IM or PO)
- *Indomethacin* 25–50 mg PO TID
- *Ibuprofen* 800 mg PO TID

Opioids (morphine, hydromorphone, tramadol) are the second choice and can also be effective in providing analgesia, but can worsen nausea and vomiting.

- A combination of IV *morphine* and ketorolac is more effective than either drug alone, and is also associated with a decrease in rescue analgesia

α-Blockers can help reduce recurrent colic if taken on a daily basis.

Hydration

Many patients present with some combination of vomiting, anorexia, and moderate to severe dehydration. As such, IV hydration should be rapidly initiated upon presentation, with a relatively rapid rate if the patient's cardiopulmonary status is amenable.

 – If high-rate infusion is not an option, 20 cc/h of normal saline has been demonstrated to be as effective as bolused hydration with 2 L of normal saline over 2 h with regard to pain perception and analgesia usage
 – There is no evidence for the use of diuretics in the treatment of acute renal colic

As vomiting and nausea are a key component leading to dehydration in patients with renal colic, appropriate therapy with an anti-emetic can be critical.

 – *Metoclopramide chloride* 0.5 mg/kg/day IV over three doses is especially effective

Medical Expulsive Therapy

Patients for whom urgent intervention is not indicated may be offered observation, with or without medical expulsive therapy (MET).

Medical expulsive therapy (MET) differs from observation in that pharmacologic agents are used to facilitate stone expulsion. These agents act by relaxing ureteral smooth muscle, either via calcium channel pumps inhibition or alpha-1 receptor blockade.

Appropriate Patient Selection

Any patient with the following symptoms requires decompression via indwelling stent or percutaneous nephrostomy tube drainage, and is not appropriate for MET

- Urine infection with concomitant urinary tract obstruction [6]
  - Temperature $\geq 38.0\ ^\circ C$
  - Leukocytosis $\geq 15,000/mL$
  - + leukocyte esterase and + nitrite (sensitivity 68–88 %)
- Urosepsis
- Intractable pain, nausea, or vomiting
- Bilateral obstructing stones or obstruction of a solitary or transplanted kidney[1]
- Obstructing ureteral calculus in a pregnant female[1]
- Inadequate renal function reserve

Patient preferences and comorbidities need also be taken into account when making a treatment decision.

---

[1] Although these may not be absolute contraindications, they should only be attempted in the most compliant patients who are amenable to extremely close (weekly) follow-up.

Medications

The mainstays of MET are *α-blockers* and *calcium channel blockers* [7].

- *Tamsulosin* 0.4 mg PO QD is the best studied medication
  - Effect has also been demonstrated for the class of α-blockers including doxazosin, terazosin, alfuzosin, and naftopidil, although these drugs have been studied less frequently
  - Meta-analysis of existing randomized controlled trials calculates the number needed to treat four patients to avoid one surgery
- *Nifedipine* 30 mg XR PO QD is the only calcium-channel blocked that has been investigated, but it has been shown to have an expulsive effect on stones <10 mm
- *Corticosteroids* at low dosages may have an effect when used in conjunction with an α-blocker but there is no evidence to support them as monotherapy

Patient Counseling

Although there is only limited data on the rates of spontaneous stone passage (unaided by MET), a meta-analysis of *ureteral stones* yielded a 68 % rate of passage for stones <5 mm in diameter (n = 224) and a 47 % rate of passage for 5–10 mm stones (n = 104), with 95 % of these stones passing within 40 days.

Opinions vary with respect to optimal management of asymptomatic renal stones. The natural history of small, nonobstructing renal stones remains poorly defined.

MET has been shown by multiple studies to accelerate spontaneous passage of ureteral stones and also of stone fragments generated with ESWL or URS. It also has been shown to decrease pain. Several factors have been shown to affect success rates [8].

- *Stone size*: stones <5 mm in size have such a high spontaneous passage rate that data on the efficacy of MET has been limited, although it does reduce analgesic requirements.
- *Stone location*: most trials include only patients with distal ureteral stones, and have demonstrated that MET facilitates expulsion in these cases. Its effect on proximal ureteral stones or renal stones is less well defined.
- *Duration of treatment*: the vast majority of stones undergoing observation pass within 40 days, but the majority of studies on MET specifically had a duration of 30 days, so some MET failures might have passed between days 31 and 40 had they been given a chance. Regardless, treatment carried beyond 40 days is unlikely to be effective.

MET cannot be recommended in children due to the lack of data, and it is unknown whether tamsulosin harms the human fetus or can be transmitted via breast milk. Patients should also be counseled that MET is an *off-label use* of these medications, and should be counseled about the attendant risks, including drug side effects.

Follow-up

Patients should be offered follow-up *within the first 14 days* of a trial of MET, and should be evaluated for hydronephrosis as well as stone position at this time ideally via US and KUB, or CT if patient or stone characteristics are not conducive (BMI, patient tolerance, stone location, etc). If this initial round of follow-up is negative for stone passage, MET may be continued so long as the patient's pain continues to be well controlled, there is no evidence of sepsis, and adequate renal functional reserve remains. Since 95 % of stones that will pass spontaneously do so within the first 40 days, treatment of patients with MET should conclude no later than 6 weeks [6].

- Patients should be instructed to *strain their urine* and report back to their urologist if they pass the stone, saving the stone for analysis

- *Intractable pain, nausea* and/or *vomiting*, and *fever* ≥38 °C should prompt re-evaluation by a physician, with fever being the most urgent indication for re-evaluation

Special Considerations

- Regardless of method of treatment, *all patients with bacteriuria should receive appropriate antibiotic therapy*
- Patients with a *kidney transplant*
  - Any unexplained deterioration, including fever or failure to thrive, should prompt consideration of a renal calculus and prompt evaluation with US or NCCT
  - Conservative treatment in these patients is only acceptable for small, asymptomatic stones in absolutely compliant patients and under close surveillance via serial serum creatinine measurement
- Patients with *neurogenic bladder*
  - Any patient with neurogenic bladder dysfunction or who has undergone urinary diversion is at higher risk for recurrent stone formation
  - These patients should therefore be managed with an eye to the long term, with special attention paid to metabolic workup, obtaining culture data for appropriate antibiosis selection, and minimization of unnecessary radiation exposure given the high likelihood of repeated imaging over the course of their disease

References

1. EAU/AUA Nephrolithiasis Guideline Panel. Guideline for the management of ureteral calculi. Baltimore (MD): American Urological Association Education and Research, Inc., Eur Assoc Urol; 2007. p. 1–61.
2. Angulo JC, Gaspar MJ, Rodriguez N, et al. The value of C-reactive protein determination in patients with renal colic to decide urgent urinary diversion. J Urol. 2010;76(2):301–6.

3. Antonelli JA, Fulgham PF, Pearle MS. Imaging in the management of ureteral calculi. Am Urol Assoc Update Ser. 2013;32(37):373.
4. Fulgham PF, Assimos DG, Pearle MS, et al. Clinical effectiveness protocols for imaging in the management of ureteral calculus disease: AUA technology assessment. J Urol. 2013;189(4):1203.
5. Bader P, Echtle D, Fonteyne V, et al. Non-traumatic acute flank pain. Guidelines on pain management. Arnhem: European Association of Urology (EAU); 2010. p. 82–90.
6. Pearle MS. Management of the acute stone event. Am Urol Assoc Update Ser. 2008;27(30):281–92.
7. Hollingsworth JM, Rogers MA, Kauffman SR, et al. Medical therapy to facilitate urinary stone passage; a meta-analysis. Lancet. 2006;368:1171–9.
8. Turk C, Knoll T, Petrik A, et al. Guidelines on urolithiasis. Arnhem: European Association of Urology (EAU); 2013. p. 17–26, 50–62.

Chapter 17
Stratifying Surgical Therapy

Vincent G. Bird, Benjamin K. Canales, and John M. Shields

Abbreviations

SWL   Shockwave lithotripsy
PCNL Percutaneous nephrolithotomy
URS   Ureteroscopy

Treatment Options for Renal Stones

There are four main surgical treatment modalities for renal stones.

- Extracorporeal shockwave lithotripsy (SWL)
- Rigid/flexible retrograde ureteroscopy (URS)
- Percutaneous nephrolithotomy (PCNL)
- Laparoscopic/open surgery

A general decision-tree algorithm of the most common of these approaches, stratified by stone size, density, and location, is presented in Fig. 17.1. Since they represent the full

---

V.G. Bird, MD (✉) • B.K. Canales, MD • J.M. Shields, MD
Department of Urology, University of Florida College of Medicine,
1600 SW Archer Road, P.O. Box 100247, Gainesville, FL 32610, USA
e-mail: Vincent.bird@urology.ufl.edu

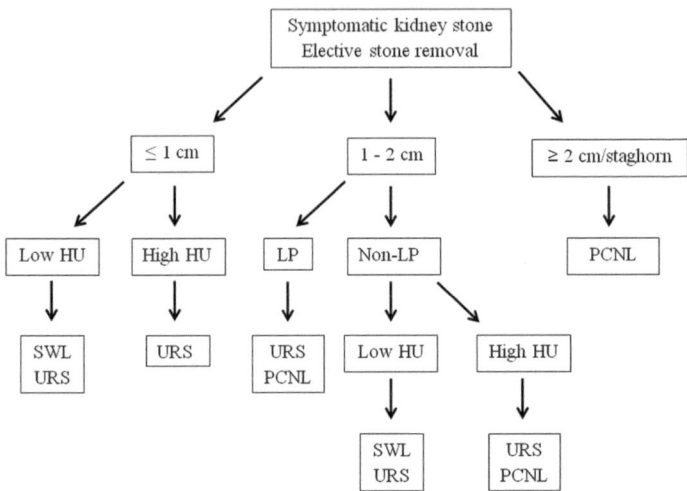

Fig. 17.1. Proposed algorithm for kidney stone management, stratified by stone size, HU (Hounsfield unit densities), and non-LP/LP (lower pole) locations

spectrum of endourologic techniques, a brief review of the principles behind these strategies is appropriate.

Extracorporeal Shockwave Lithotripsy

SWL consists of transmission of high-energy shock waves, created by an energy source, such as electrohydraulic, electromagnetic, and others, through the patient. The shockwave can be focused on the stone in question using an acoustic lens and transmitted through water or a membrane in contact with the patient. When these shock waves approach the calculus and thus pass through two different acoustic mediums, energy is released, resulting in fragmentation of the calculus due to a disruption in the internal structure of the stone. This can be achieved with the aid of fluoroscopy or ultrasound guidance as a means to target the exact location of the calculus, and thus focus the acoustic waves precisely on the calculus. SWL is non-invasive, can be delivered with or without general anesthesia, and can be done on an outpatient basis. Success rates vary when compared to alternative modalities, however, in a comparison study between SWL, URS, and PCNL, single treatment rates were significantly better in patients who underwent PCNL and URS when compared to SWL [1]. SWL was shown to necessitate repeated treatments in order to match the efficacies of PCNL and URS [1, 2].

SWL has reduced effectiveness in patients who are more obese, as well as patients with hard stones and stones which are large or involve complex anatomy. Impacted ureteral and/or lower pole stones can prove more difficult to clear and may benefit from pre-SWL manipulation to an upper or midpolar location; ureteral stent placement may also be performed during this setting to facilitate passage of stone fragments. Post-procedural positioning exercises may also improve clearance. In rare circumstances, SWL is shown to have potential consequences including significant hemorrhage from the kidney, spleen, and liver. Its relationship to diabetes mellitus and hypertension is less certain and has been a subject of contention [2, 3]. Nonetheless, due to its non-invasive nature and minimal anesthesia requirements, SWL is often administered as a first line of treatment for stones less than 2 cm.

Ureteroscopy

Advances in fiber optics and digital imaging as well as improvements with ancillary equipment have led to significant progress in the endoscopic management of ureteral and renal stones. Ureteroscopy (URS) consists of retrograde passage of an endoscope per urethra and upward through to the affected ureter and kidney allowing access to the calculus as well as delivery of instruments such as guidewires, balloon dilators, laser fibers, and baskets. This is relatively non-invasive but does warrant spinal or general anesthesia. A meta-analysis reviewing seven large randomized controlled trials including 1,205 patients demonstrated that ureteroscopic management of ureteral and renal stones, when compared to SWL, achieved a higher stone-free rate after treatment and lower need for retreatment [4]. As such, URS is considered treatment of choice for most ureteral and renal calculi. However, URS is associated with a higher procedure-related complication rate and longer hospital stays. Rigid ureteroscopes are reserved for more distal ureteral stones whereas flexible ureteroscopes, with their ability to deflect up to 300° in some models, can reach the extremes of renal poles as well as negotiate otherwise difficult to access anatomic variants of renal calices. As the deflection capabilities can be reduced significantly once the working channel is utilized, it may help to move the calculus to a more accessible calyx.

Improved endoscopic equipment has also facilitated this procedure greatly with improved stone-free rates. Ureteral stents when placed prior to ureteroscopic treatment for urinary lithiasis were shown to be associated with higher stone-free rates [5]. Ureteral access sheaths allow repetitive passage of ureteroscopes to and from the renal pelvis while minimizing trauma to the urothelium. Ureteral access sheaths also allow continuous flow of irrigation fluid thereby improving visualization and facilitating a low-pressure system. While flexible electrohydraulic lithotripters are available for both rigid and flexible ureteroscopes, laser lithotripsy remains the preferred method of choice for lithotripsy in most first-world centers; the most efficient laser system being the Ho:YAG system, due to its rapid absorption in water and minimal tissue penetration. There exists an increasing array of basketing and grasping instruments available to the surgeon. While graspers allow for easier release of the stone if removal becomes difficult, extraction usually takes longer than when using baskets. With regard to guidewires, it is recommended to leave a safety wire in place, as in the case of ureteral injury access may be lost otherwise. Ureteral stent placement over the wire will also obviate the need for a percutaneous nephrostomy tube to be placed for urinary drainage.

17. Stratifying Surgical Therapy 153

Percutaneous Nephrolithotomy

PCNL involves direct passage of an endoscope percutaneously into the kidney. Access is achieved under fluoroscopic or ultrasonic guidance or combined endoscopic/radiographic imaging techniques. With the patient in either a prone or supine position, the kidney is located using anatomical markings as a rough guide; a posterior approach below the 12th rib is preferred to avoid the pleura as well as the intercostal vessels and nerve. Access via a posterior calyx is preferred rather than the renal pelvis so as to avoid the posterior branches of the renal artery which runs along the renal pelvis. A percutaneous puncture is done with a needle followed by injection of contrast to reveal the intrarenal anatomy. This can be done as an outpatient procedure in an angiography suite or during the same setting of the PCNL. Cystoscopy and placement of a ureteral catheter with retrograde injection of contrast can dramatically aid in localizing and accessing the kidney prior to placement of the percutaneous needle.

Once access has been obtained, and a guide wire can be advanced in an antegrade fashion to maintain access as well as to allow passage of dilators in order to expand the tract; sequential dilators or a balloon dilator can be used. Speculation regarding the safety, efficacy, and long-term sequelae of either method has been put forth, but no large long-term studies have proven either method to be superior. Once access and dilation is achieved, with a working sheath in place, a rigid or flexible nephroscope can be passed along with a variety of lithotripters: laser, pneumatic, ultrasonic, or a combined pneumatic/ultrasonic lithotripter. Calculi can then be removed in fairly large sizes as the access sheaths can be as large as 30 Fr. Antegrade access to the ureter can be achieved depending on ureteral diameter.

Bleeding can obstruct visibility and often requires termination of the procedure with placement of a nephrostomy tube and a return to the operating room at a later date. Anatomical limitations can also make it difficult or impossible to access calyces with a narrow infundibulum or with entrances at acute angles to the tract. In these cases, a second and sometimes third access tract is required to obtain complete stone clearance. A combined retrograde approach is also an option. Critical to successful PCNL is optimal positioning of the nephrostomy tract for complete stone removal and thus if a radiologist is placing the nephrostomy tube prior to the PCNL, good communication between the urologist and the radiologist is paramount.

A nephrostomy is often left in place along with a ureteral stent to allow for maximal drainage, however a number of studies have shown that leaving the patient without a nephrostomy tube or "tubeless" is often equally safe and effective [6].

Due to the more invasive nature of PCNL, there is a greater risk for complications, although rare, when compared to less invasive endoscopic techniques. These include bleeding, perforation of the large bowel, pneumo/hydro/hemo-thorax, and arteriovenous fistula development post-operatively. In a large multicenter study of 1,448 patients with large kidney stones, complications, longer operative times, fever, and increased rates of transfusion were seen in patients who had larger (4–6 cm) kidney stones compared to those with smaller (2–3 cm) kidney stones [7].

PCNL generally offers very high stone-free rates, which can be attributed to the shorter distance to traverse as well as introduction of a relatively large working sheath, allowing for larger and more effective instruments, and removal of larger stone fragments. Though this procedure regularly requires general anesthesia and increased analgesia, for patients with a larger stone burden greater than 2 cm or staghorn calculi, a percutaneous approach is preferred. Success rates are similar to those of open surgery, while decreasing the length hospital stay by 60 %. Patients may be able to work within one week after PCNL, as compared to greater than three weeks after open renal surgery. PCNL has also been shown to be 40 % less expensive when compared to open surgery [8].

Open/Laparoscopic Nephrolithotomy

With the arrival of advanced endoscopic techniques, open/laparoscopic nephrolithotomy is performed less commonly. However, open/laparoscopic surgery still plays a significant role for a small number of patients; namely, patients with complex large volume stones and/or complex renal anatomy, particularly large calculi in anterior caliceal diverticula. Open/laparoscopic surgery for renal stones may also be considered for patients with abnormal body habitus, such as obesity or kyphosis, as well as patients who will most likely require multiple attempts and tracts placed for PCNL, and who also want only one attempt at surgery to be performed. Patients who present with renal calculi and concomitant ureteropelvic junction obstruction may also be considered for open/laparoscopic surgery in order to address both the obstruction and the renal calculi, as well as stones found in a non-functioning kidney [9]. With advances in laparoscopic and robotic techniques, many of these procedures can now be done through a minimally invasive approach.

Complications specific to open stone surgery include wound infection, hernia, increased risk of transfusion, and longer hospital stay when compared to endoscopic removal. Perinephric scarring resulting from open/laparoscopic surgery may make subsequent surgeries more difficult if necessary. Overall, since the advent and evolution of SWL, PCNL, endoscopic equipment, and techniques, the need for open stone surgery has been greatly reduced.

Determining Treatment Modality

A number of factors, summarized in Table 17.1, play a role in determining the best modality of treatment of renal stones and are briefly reviewed.

TABLE 17.1 Success rates, risks, and contraindications for renal stone procedures

Location/procedure	Stone size indications (cm)	Success rates (%)	Risks	Absolute and relative contraindications
Non-LP SWL	≤1.5	50–70	Steinstrasse/obstruction 2–5 %; UTI 1–2 %; Hematoma 2 %; Sepsis 1–2 %; Fever 2 %; ? diabetes risk	Coagulopathy, pregnancy, obesity (>12 cm SSD), obstruction, renal anomalies, cysteine, or calcium oxalate monohydrate composition, dense stones (HU > 1,000); radiolucent stones
LP SWL	≤1	50		
Non-LP URS	<2	60–80	Stent pain 40 %, UTI 5 %; Sepsis 1 %; Ureteral injury 5 % (minor), 0.1 % (major)	Bladder reconstruction, ileal conduit, renal transplantation, ureteral stricture, or ureteral pathology
LP URS	≤1.5	50–60		
Non-LP PCNL	>2	80–95	Blood transfusion 5 %; sepsis 2–5 %; chest tube placement 1 %; renal arterial embolization 1 %	Coagulopathy, pregnancy, high pulmonary risk, inability to tolerate prone position, unstable prone airway
LP PCNL	≥1.5	70–80		

Key: LP lower pole, *SWL* shock wave lithotripsy, *URS* ureteroscopy, *PCNL* percutaneous nephrolithotomy, *UTI* urinary tract infection, *SSD* skin to stone distance

Size

For stones less than 2 cm, SWL or URS is favored. For stones greater than 2 cm, SWL may result in a trail of stone fragments which line the ureter and has been suitably named "Steinstrasse" (German for "street of stone"). Significant obstruction may also result from this process. For stones greater than 2 cm, PCNL is favored over URS, as PCNL can often clear stones with a fewer number of procedures. For much larger stones, such as staghorn calculi or stones occupying multiple, distant, hard to reach calyces, PCNL is preferred. However open/laparoscopic surgery may also be utilized in rare specific circumstances.

Location

Lower pole stones are often best managed with URS or PCNL, as SWL tends to result in stone fragments which are reluctant to drain by gravity and urine flow. Often times the lower pole stone can be repositioned to the renal pelvis or an upper or middle calyx with URS in order to facilitate treatment without excessive torquing and deflection of the ureteroscope. Percutaneous access via an upper calyx will allow a more direct approach toward the lower calyx versus a middle calyx access.

Stone Composition

Stone composition can be determined by chemical analysis, by history, or radiographic appearance. Calcium oxalate dihydrate and uric acid calculi tend to be easily degraded by SWL, whereas cystine, pure calcium phosphate (i.e., Brushite), and calcium oxalate monohydrate may be refractory to SWL and better suited to laser, pneumatic, or ultrasonic lithotripsy.

Anatomical

Factors such as morbid obesity may in particular circumstances require open or laparoscopic approach, as a percutaneous approach may not prove to be as efficacious or practical due to the increased body mass. This is also true for patients with kyphosis or scoliosis. Pregnancy also plays a significant role as pregnant women are generally best not exposed to ionizing radiation, i.e., fluoroscopy, particularly during the first and second trimester. In these cases URS under ultrasound guidance is preferred. There is also the option of placement of an internal stent and deferment of surgery until delivery of the fetus.

Conclusion

As with any surgical procedure, the risks and benefits should be carefully reviewed with the patient prior to selection of appropriate therapy. The miniaturization of endoscopic equipment and improved imaging technologies will undoubtedly march us toward better techniques to destroy and removal of renal calculi. As such, the ultimate goals of these advances are to reduce the morbidity and mortality associated with current treatment options, all the while improving stone-free rates as well as post-operative patient symptoms and quality of life.

References

1. Wiesenthal JD, Ghiculete D, D'A Honey RJ, Pace KT. A comparison of treatment modalities for renal calculi between 100 and 300 mm^2: are shockwave lithotripsy, ureteroscopy, and percutaneous nephrolithotomy equivalent? J Endourol. 2011;25(3):481–5.
2. Gupta M, Bolton DM, Irby 3rd P, Hubner W, Wolf Jr JS, Hattner RS, et al. The effect of newer generation lithotripsy upon renal function assessed by nuclear scintigraphy. J Urol. 1995;154(3): 947–50.

3. Krambeck AE, Gettman MT, Rohlinger AL, Lohse CM, Patterson DE, Segura JW. Diabetes mellitus and hypertension associated with shock wave lithotripsy of renal and proximal ureteral stones at 19 years of followup. J Urol. 2006;175(5):1742–7.
4. Aboumarzouk OM, Kata SG, Keeley FX, McClinton S, Nabi G. Extracorporeal shock wave lithotripsy (ESWL) versus ureteroscopic management for ureteric calculi. Cochrane Database Syst Rev. 2012;5, CD006029.
5. Shields JM, Bird VG, Graves R, Gomez-Marin O. Impact of preoperative ureteral stenting on outcome of ureteroscopic treatment for urinary lithiasis. J Urol. 2009;182(6):2768–74.
6. Akman T, Binbay M, Yuruk E, Sari E, Seyrek M, Kaba M, et al. Tubeless procedure is most important factor in reducing length of hospitalization after percutaneous nephrolithotomy: result of univariable and multivariable models. Urology. 2011;77(2): 299–304.
7. Xue W, Pacik D, Boellaard W, Breda A, Botoca M, Raasweiller J, Van Cleynenbreugel B, et al. Management of single large non-staghorn renal stones in the CROES PCNL global study. J Urol. 2012;187(4):1293–7.
8. Preminger GM, Clayman RV, Hardeman SW, Franklin J, Curry T, Peters PC. Percutaneous nephrolithotomy vs. open surgery for renal calculi. A comparative study. JAMA. 1985;254(8):1054–8.
9. Segura JW, Preminger GM, Assimos DG, Dretler SP, Kahn RI, Lingeman JE, et al. Nephrolithiasis clinical guidelines panel summary report on the management of staghorn calculi. The American urological association nephrolithiasis clinical guidelines panel. J Urol. 1994;151(6):1648–51.

Index

A
Acetohydroxamic acid, 106
Acidic urine, 82
Acute renal colic. *See* Renal colic, acute
Alanine-glyoxylate aminotransferase (AGXT), 65–66
Alkali citrate preparations, 56
Alkaline salt therapy, 81
Alkali therapy, hypercalciuria
  adverse effects, 44
  mechanism of action, 43
  medications, 43–44
α-blockers, 142, 144
Alpha-mercapto-propionylglycine, 94
American Urological Association (AUA) guidelines, kidney stone management, 113, 114
Amiloride, 45
Amorphous urinary crystals, 117
Anatrophic nephrolithotomy, 107–108
Antibiotics, struvite stones, 105
Anti-nutrient. *See* Oxalate
Arachadonic acid (AA), 34

Asymptomatic stones
  follow-up strategies, 133
  history, 131–132
  percutaneous nephrolithotomy, 134
  residual fragments, 132
  shockwave lithotripsy, 133–134
  special groups, 134–135
  treatment, 133–134

B
Basic metabolic panel (BMP), 21
Bisphosphonates, hypercalciuria, 46
Body mass index (BMI) calculation, 10
Bowel disease, 82
Brushite urinary crystals, 117

C
Calcium oxalate monohydrate urinary crystals, 117
Calcium oxalate supersaturation, 64
Captopril, 95
Carbonate apatite, 102, 103, 106
Chlorthalidone, 42

Chronic diarrhea, 16, 51
Citrate therapy, 56–59
Citric acid, 52, 53, 58
Coffin-lid shaped urinary crystals, 117
Cranberry juice, struvite stone prevention, 104
Cyanide-nitroprusside test, 92
Cystine capacity, 93, 95
Cystine stones
  management, 25
  sodium intake, 12
  ultrasound, 93
Cystinuria
  adults and children, 91
  $B^{0,+}$ AT subunit, 91
  cyanide-nitroprusside test, 92, 93
  definition, 91
  diagnosis, 92
  fluid intakes, 93–94
  genetic mutations, 92
  24-h cystine excretion analysis, 93
  increasing urine pH, 94
  non-type 1 carriers, 92
  proximal tubular cystine transporter system, 91
  random amino acid analysis, 93
  rBAT subunit, 91
  SLC3A1, 92
  SLC7A9, 92
  treatment, 96
  type I, 92
  urine collections, 95
  vegetarian diet, 94

D
Diclofenac, 141
Digital tomosynthesis (DT), 127–128
$_D$-penicillamine, 94
Dysbiosis, 69

E
Eicosapentaenoic acid (EPA), 34
EQUIL2 formula, 119

F
Fish oil
  hypercalciuria, 33–34
  role, 70, 71

G
Gastrointestinal (GI) tract
  bacterial oxalate degradation, 68–69
  calcium and magnesium content, 67–68
  controlling oxalate absorption, 66–68
  fat malabsorption, 70
  oxalate intake, 69–70
Gravel/colic syndrome, 84

H
HCTZ. *See* Hydrochlorothiazide (HCTZ)
Hexagonal urinary crystals, 117
High risk stone formers, 118
Hounsfield unit count, 83
Hydrochlorothiazide (HCTZ), 41, 42
Hypercalciuria
  alkali therapy
    adverse effects, 44
    mechanism of action, 43
    medications, 43–44
  amiloride, 45
  bisphosphonates, 46
  complications, 39
  definition, 37
  diagnosis, 39
  etiology, 38
  neutral phosphates
    adverse effects, 45

efficacy, 44–45
mechanism of action, 44
nutrition management
 alcohol and caffeine, 33
 carbohydrate diet intake, 33
 dietary acid load, 31–32
 dietary calcium, 29–30
 dietary sodium, 30–31
 fiber intake, 32
 fish oil, 33–34
 weight loss, 33
periodic monitoring, 45–46
thiazide diuretics
 adverse effects, 42–43
 efficacy, 41
 mechanism of action, 41
 medications, 42
treatment, 40–41
 duration, 45
Hyperoxaluria
 idiopathic, 66
 primary, 65, 66
 vitamin B6 deficiency, 66
Hypocitraturia
 citrate intake, 52–53
 definition, 49, 55
 diarrhea, 51–52
 high dietary acid load, 50
 juices and juice products, 52–53
 low carbohydrate diets, 50
 low potassium intake, 50–51
 magnesium intake, 52
 malabsorption, 51–52
 medical nutrition therapy, 49
 prevalence, 55
Hypokalemia, 15, 43, 50, 57, 115

I
Ibuprofen, 142
Indapamide, 42
Indomethacin, 142
Intestinal dysfunction, prototype, 82

K
Ketorolac, 142

L
Livingston equation, 10

M
Medical expulsive therapy (MET)
 bacteriuria patients, 146
 corticosteroids, 144
 follow-up, 145–146
 kidney transplant patients, 146
 neurogenic bladder patients, 146
 nifedipine, 144
 patient counseling, 144–145
 patient selection, 143
 spontaneous ureteral stone passage, 144
 tamsulosin, 144
Medical nutrition therapy (MNT), 49
MET. *See* Medical expulsive therapy (MET)
Metabolic work-up, 4–5
Mifflin St. Jeor equation, 10

N
NCCT. *See* Non-contrast computed tomography (NCCT)
Nephrectomy, struvite stones, 107
Nephrolithiasis
 non-contrast computed tomography, 124
 plain abdominal radiography, 126
Neutral phosphates, hypercalciuria
 adverse effects, 45
 efficacy, 44–45
 mechanism of action, 44

Non-contrast computed tomography (NCCT)
  acute renal colic, 141
  cost, 125
  drawbacks, 124
  flank pain, 141
  low dose, 124–125
  sensitivity and specificity, 124
Nutrition guidelines
  BMI calculation, 10
  calcium intake, 12–13
  energy balance, 10
  fluid intake, 11–12
  24-h urine collection, 9
  Livingston equation, 10
  Mifflin St. Jeor equation, 10
  obesity, 10
  resting metabolic rate, 10
  urinary citrate
    chronic diarrhea, 15
    dietary intake of citrate, 13–14
    hypokalemia, 15
    potassium intake, 15
    potential renal acid load, 14–15
Nutrition management
  hyperoxaluria (*see* Hyperoxaluria)
  hypocitraturia, 49–54

O
Obesity, 10
Omega-3 fatty acids, 33–34
Open/laparoscopic nephrolithotomy, 155
Open struvite stone surgery, 107–108
Opioids, 142
Oxalate, 63
  biosynthesis control, 65–66
  calcium oxalate supersaturation, 64
  gastrointestinal tract
    absorption control, 66–68
    concentration, 68–70

P
Penicillamine, 95
Percutaneous nephrolithotomy (PCNL)
  asymptomatic stones, 134
  complications, 154
  description, 153–154
  high stone-free rates, 154
  struvite stones, 107
Plain abdominal radiography (KUB)
  advantages, 126
  disadvantages, 126–127
  radiation dose, 126
  sensitivity and specificity, 126
  and tomograms, 127
Plant-based purines, 76
Potassium citrate, 85–87
  benefit, 57
  cystine excretion, 94
  doses, 43
  dosing, 58, 59
  gastrointestinal side effects, 58
  liquid preparations, 57, 58
  lower rates of stone recurrence, 56, 57
  sodium, 44
  tablet forms, 57
  usage, 43
Potassium magnesium citrate, 44, 56
Potential renal acid load (PRAL), 14–15, 50, 51
  of foods, 32
  merits, 78
  negative values, 78
  positive values, 77–78
Primary hyperparathyroidism, 115, 116
Probenecid, 83
Prostaglandin E2 (PGE2), 34
Pyridoxine, 65, 66

R

Recurrent calcium nephrolithiasis, 56, 59
Recurrent stone former
  creatinine values, 119
  follow-up, 113, 114
  24-h urine collection, 118–120
  imaging studies, 123–129
  laboratory evaluation, 113
  metabolic testing, 118
  radiation exposure and imaging cost, 123–124
  serum testing, 114–116
  stone analysis, 116–118
  supersaturation index, 119
  urinalysis, 116
Renacidin, 106
Renal colic, acute
  analgesia, 141–142
  definition, 139
  differential diagnosis
    acute uncomplicated pyelonephritis, 139
    renal infarction and/or renal vein thrombosis, 139
    renal papillary necrosis, 140
    renal/ureteral stone, 139
    spontaneous renal hemorrhage, 140
    testicular torsion, 140
    uretero-pelvic junction obstruction, 140
  hydration, 142
  lab work, 140
  medical expulsive therapy, 143–146
  non-contrast enhanced computed tomography, 141
Renal stones, surgical treatment
  decision-tree algorithm, 149, 150
  extracorporeal shockwave lithotripsy, 150–151
  morbid obesity, 158
  open/laparoscopic nephrolithotomy, 155
  percutaneous nephrolithotomy, 153–154
  pregnancy, 158
  stone composition, 157
  stone size and location, 157
  success rates, risks, and contraindications, 155, 156
  ureteroscopy, 151–152
Renal ultrasound (RUS)
  advantages, 126
  cost, 126
  limitations, 125
Residual fragments, 132
Resting metabolic rate (RMR), 10
RUS. *See* Renal ultrasound (RUS)

S

Secondary hyperparathyroidism, 116
Serum tests
  basic blood chemistry, 21
  hyperparathyroidism and serum calcium evaluation, 21, 23
  indications, 19
  kidney stone formers, 20–21
  parathyroid axis, 23
  serum lab tests and utility, 21, 22
Shockwave lithotripsy (SWL)
  asymptomatic stones, 133–134
  description, 150–151
  minimal anesthesia requirements, 151
  non-invasive nature, 151
  struvite stones, 107
Small bowel resection, Crohn's disease, 82
Sodium bicarbonate, 85–87
Sodium citrate, 58
Sodium-potassium citrate treatment, 56, 57

Staghorn calculi
  percutaneous nephrolithotomy, 107, 154, 157
  struvite stones, 101
Stone recurrence
  calcium oxalate stones, 5
  metabolic work-up, 4–5
  risk factors, 4
  statistics, 3–4
  supersaturation, 5–6
  urinary citrate, 5
Struvite stones
  antibiotics, 105
  composition, 101
  diagnostic testing, 103
  dissolution therapy, 106
  epidemiology, 101–102
  etiology, 102
  microbiological culture, 103
  nephrectomy, 107
  open stone surgery, 107
  percutaneous nephrolithotomy, 107
  risk factors, 102
  shockwave lithotripsy, 107
  treatment and prevention, 103–104
  urease inhibitors, 105–106
  urease-producing bacteria, 103
  ureteroscopy, 107
  urine pH, 103
Suby's G solution, 106
Supersaturation index, 119
SWL. *See* Shockwave lithotripsy (SWL)

T

Thiazide diuretics, hypercalciuria
  adverse effects, 42–43
  efficacy, 41
  mechanism of action, 41
  medications, 42
Tiopronin, 94, 95
Tomograms, 127

U

Ultrasound
  cystine stones, 93
  renal, 125–126
Ureteroscopy (URS), 96
  description, 151–152
  struvite stones, 107
Uric acid stones
  catabolic states and chemotherapy, 83
  clinical presentations, 84
  dehydration, 83
  diagnosis, 83–84
  dissolving and prevention, 85–86
  high protein diet, 83
  ileostomy patients, 82
  intermittent *vs.* continuous therapy, 86–87
  low urinary pH, 81
  nutrition management
    alcohol consumption, 76–77
    fluid intakes, 75
    fructose intake, 78
    metabolic syndrome, 78, 79
    obesity, 78, 79
    proteins, 76
    purines, 76
    type 2 diabetes mellitus, 78, 79
    urine acidity, 77–78
  pH values, 84
  potassium, advantages, 85
  rapid weight loss, 83
  sodium bicarbonate, 85–86
  ureteral obstruction, 84
  uricosuric drugs, 83
Uric acid urinary crystals, 117
Uricosuric drugs, 83
Urinary calcium excretion, 39
Urinary citrate
  acidosis, 51
  alkali-poor foods, 50
  calcium nephrolithiasis, 49
  calcium stone disease, 55
  chronic diarrhea, 15

dietary intake of citrate, 13–14
excretion, 55–56
low carbohydrate diets, 50
low potassium intake and
 urinary potassium, 50, 51
oral magnesium, 52
potassium intake, 15
potential renal acid load, 14–15
stone recurrence, 5
therapy, 56–59
Urinary oxalate
 dietary measures/
  recommendations, 64–65
 excretion, 64
 nutritional management,
  64–65
 probiotic supplements, 69
24-hour Urine test
 cystine screening, 25
 indications, 19
 patient evaluation, 24, 25
Urolithiasis
 adverse effects of
  medications, 115
 recurrent cystine urolithiasis
  patients, 120

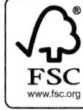

MIX
Papier aus verantwortungsvollen Quellen
Paper from responsible sources
FSC® C105338

If you have any concerns about our products,
you can contact us on
ProductSafety@springernature.com

In case Publisher is established outside the EU,
the EU authorized representative is:
**Springer Nature Customer Service Center GmbH
Europaplatz 3, 69115 Heidelberg, Germany**

Printed by Libri Plureos GmbH
in Hamburg, Germany